# A HANDBOOK OF MITRAL VALVE DISEASE

## Alok Ranjan

MD, DNB, MRCP (UK), DM (Card.)
Sr. Consultant - Cardiology
Wockhardt Hospitals
India

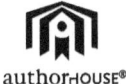

authorHOUSE®

AuthorHouse™
1663 Liberty Drive
Bloomington, IN 47403
www.authorhouse.com
Phone: 1-800-839-8640

Illustrations by Dr. Rita Sinha

Published by AuthorHouse    05/18/2013

ISBN: 978-1-4817-3554-4 (sc)
ISBN: 978-1-4817-3553-7 (hc)
ISBN: 978-1-4817-3552-0 (e)

Library of Congress Control Number: 2013906424

# Disclaimer

Medicine is a constantly changing science. New research findings necessitate continual changes in disease concept and its management. The author and publisher of this handbook have used reasonable efforts to provide up-to-date, accurate information that is within generally accepted medical standards at the time of publication. However, as medical science is ever evolving, and human error is always possible, the author and publisher (or any other involved parties) do not guarantee total accuracy or comprehensiveness of the information in this handbook, and they are not responsible for omissions, errors, or the results of using this information. The reader should confirm the accuracy of the information in this handbook from other sources. In particular, all drug doses, indications, and contraindications should be confirmed in package inserts.

The author has made every effort to trace the copyright holders for borrowed material. If he has inadvertently overlooked any, he will be pleased to make necessary arrangement at the first opportunity.

Dedicated to persons who have inspired me
with their advice, actions, teachings and affection
to strive for success in life.

They are; Mr. B B Ram, Dr. (Mrs.) Sarla Ram (grandparents),
Mr. Binod Chandra, Mr. J N Singh, Mr. Manoj Chandra (Uncles),
Mr. Prabhat Ranjan (Brother) and Dr. (Mrs.) Rita Sinha (Sister).

People might not always remember every person that they crossed
paths with in the past, but they usually remember the ones that shined
positive light on their negativity, and showed them the path that
guarantees self-fulfillment.
- **Edmond Mbiaka**

# Contents

# Mitral Stenosis

# Introduction

Mitral stenosis is due to thickening and immobility of the mitral valve leaflets, resulting in obstruction in blood flow from the left atrium to the left ventricle. The mitral valve leaflets are thickened and the commissures are fused along with thickening and shortening of the chordae tendineae. This mechanical obstruction leads to increases in pressure within the left atrium, pulmonary vasculature, and right side of the heart; in comparison, the left ventricle is unaffected if there is pure mitral stenosis.

Mitral stenosis is almost always the result of rheumatic fever. The normal area of the mitral valve orifice is 4-6 sq. cm. When this orifice is reduced to 2 sq.cm, increased left atrial pressure (LAP) is necessary for normal transmitral flow. Severe MS occurs when the opening is reduced to 1 sq. cm. When the valve area is reduced to less than 2 sq. cm., symptoms develop. It starts as dyspnea on exertion and it gradually progresses as the severity of stenosis increases. Progressive disease can lead to significant symptoms and serious complications (eg, pulmonary edema, systemic embolism, pulmonary hypertension and right heart failure), if the disease is allowed to follow its natural course.

Echocardiography is the gold standard method for detection and assessment of severity of mitral stenosis.

Mitral stenosis is a disabling and eventually lethal disease. It is a leading cause of congestive heart failure in developing countries. Although medical therapy can relieve symptoms, it does not affect the

3

obstruction to flow. As a result, interventions either percutaneous [percutaneous balloon mitral valvotomy (PBMV)] or surgical (closed or open commissurotomy and valve replacement) are required to treat patients with severe mitral stenosis.

# MS: Etiology

Most common cause is rheumatic heart disease
Rare Causes:
>Congenital
>Systemic lupus erythematosus
>Rheumatoid Arthritis
>Malignant Carcinoid
>Mitral annular Calcification
>Methysergide therapy
>Infective endocarditis
>Others; Mucopolysaccharidosis, Gout and Whipple's disease

Characteristics of RHD:

Mitral valve is the most common valve to be affected by rheumatic process
25% of RHD patients have pure or predominant MS
Another 40% RHD patients have mixed presentation i.e., MS with mitral regurgitation (MR)

Rheumatic MS shows female preponderance: M: F = 2: 3

The onset of MS after ARF in Indians is very short as compared to western population. Although it takes 10-20 years to develop MS after RF infection in western countries, the progression is more rapid in developing nations. Roy et al reported a latent period as short as 2 yrs and the shortest period reported is 6 months by Nair et al in Indian studies.

# Pathophysiology: Rheumatic MS

Pathophysiology—Rheumatic fever results in a number of pathological changes affecting the mitral valve apparatus, one or all of which may be present:

  Fusion of the leaflet commissures

  Thickening, fibrosis, and calcification of the leaflet cusps

  Thickening, fusion and shortening of the chordae tendineae

  These changes become progressive over time and result in a stenotic mitral valve which is funnel shaped, often called "fish mouthed".

Physiological changes:

  Stage I:

  **Increase in left atrial pressure** (LAP): 3 basic features are

    Reduction in MVA

    Progressive increase in diastolic transmitral gradient

    Elevation of left atrial pressure

    The normal mitral valve orifice has a cross sectional area of 4 to 6 cm2. When the orifice is reduced to 2.5 cm2, mitral stenosis is mild and there is a small diastolic gradient between the left atrium and ventricle. This increase in LAP is due to the obstruction to mitral flow and is required to maintain adequate LV filling. With mild to moderate mitral stenosis, these abnormalities are often only apparent with exercise or other conditions that increase heart rate; they eventually are seen at rest as the severity of the stenosis increases. An orifice area of $\leq 1$ cm$^2$ is considered to represent severe mitral stenosis, and is associated with a significant pressure gradient which is necessary to maintain adequate filling of the left ventricle.

The rate of progressive mitral valve narrowing varies and cannot be predicted by the initial mitral valve area or transmitral gradient. Leaflet stiffening and fibrosis are exacerbated over time by increased flow turbulence.

Stage 2:

**Passive increase in pulmonary venous pressure**: The basic features are

Increased pulmonary venous pressure

Distension of pulmonary veins/capillaries

Pulmonary congestion and edema

The increase in LAP is reflected backwards, causing an increase in pulmonary venous and capillary pressures. This leads to pulmonary venous and capillary distension. Symptoms and signs of pulmonary congestion are apparent now and if the pulmonary venous pressure exceeds 30 mm Hg, pulmonary edema develops. With severe mitral stenosis, these changes are present even at rest.

Stage 3:

**Development of pulmonary arterial hypertension**

Pulmonary hypertension is a common complication of more advanced MS

Several factors contribute to the development of pulmonary hypertension in this setting:

Passive backward transmission of the elevated left atrial pressure (Stage 2)

Pulmonary artery and arteriole vasoconstriction due to the elevated pulmonary venous pressures (reactive pulmonary hypertension; **'second stenosis' of MS**)

Hypertrophy of the pulmonary artery muscular layer as a result of the increased pressure

Organic obliterative changes in the pulmonary vascular bed due to the chronically elevated pressures

Reactive pulmonary hypertension is rare unless mitral stenosis is severe enough to cause a pulmonary capillary pressure at rest of at least 20-25 mm Hg. After this level, increase in PA pressure is no longer passive and it rises out of proportion to pulmonary capillary wedge pressure. The reason why reactive pulmonary hypertension does not develop in all patients with severe mitral stenosis is not known.

Stage 4:
**Right heart dysfunction**

Pulmonary hypertension eventually leads to right ventricular hypertrophy and enlargement, tricuspid regurgitation, increased right atrial pressure, and the development of right-sided congestive heart failure. Right heart dysfunction can progress independent of the degree of mitral stenosis at this stage.

# Hemodynamics in MS

As valve area decreases, hemodynamic perturbations become more significant. As valve area decreases to less than 2 cm$^2$, an increase in left atrial pressure is necessary for normal transmitral flow to occur. Significant symptomatic MS develops when the MVA falls to less than 1.4 cm$^2$. At valve areas less than 1 cm$^2$, a LAP of 25 mm Hg is required to maintain a normal cardiac output.

With pure mitral stenosis, the left ventricular systolic and diastolic pressures are usually normal. However, when the stenosis is very severe, there may be a decrease in left ventricular filling and end-diastolic volume (or preload) which will cause a reduction in stroke volume and cardiac output.

Summary of Hemodynamic changes:

LAP:
    Increased
    Mean: Increased (+)
    'a' wave: Greatly increased (++)
LVEDP:
    Normal
    Increased if associated with
        MR

CAD

AV disease

Hypertension

PAWP

   High

PAP

   High

      If PAP is more than 10 mm Hg than LA (mean)

         Suggestive of PVOD (Second stenosis of MS) or reactive pulmonary hypertension due to arteriolar constriction

RVSP

   If > 70 mm Hg

      Associated with raised RVEDP and increase in mean JVP

| Severity of MS | MVA (cm$^2$) | LAP (mm of Hg) |
|---|---|---|
| Minimal | > 2.5 | Normal |
| Mild | 1.4-2.5 | 10-12 |
| Moderate | 1.0-1.4 | 12-17 |
| Severe | <1.0 | > 18 |
| Critical | **<0.7** | >20-25 |

# Clinical Features of MS

## Symptoms

Dyspnea:
> Occurs due to reduced compliance of the lungs and due to the decrease in vital capacity resulting from vascular congestion and interstitial edema.
>> Dyspnea initially occurs with any condition that causes an increase in blood flow across the mitral valve or reduces the time for such blood flow to occur (i.e., diminishes the duration of diastole).
>>
>> As the degree of MS increases, dyspnea occurs with very little effort and **orthopnea** may also occur. A common complaint at this time is fatigue due to the reduction in cardiac output (Compared to MR, it is a late symptom)

Cough:  Occurs due to pulmonary congestion.

Palpitations
> Atrial arrhythmias

Chest pain:  Seen in 15 % cases

Patients with MS infrequently experience chest pain (often resembles angina)

Most commonly the result of pulmonary hypertension and right ventricular hypertrophy

Rarely due to underlying coronary artery disease or a coronary artery embolism

An atrial tachyarrhythmia with left atrial and pulmonary vascular distension is another cause of intermittent chest pain in MS

Paroxysmal nocturnal dyspnea (PND): Reasons for PND are:
Absorption of edema fluid with increase in RV output overfilling the lungs

Diminished sympathetic drive of sleep decreasing LV contractility

Sleep induced dreams with the attendant increase in emotional activity and sinus tachycardia

Nocturnal arrhythmias

Pulmonary edema: When pulmonary capillary pressure exceeds tissue oncotic pressure (about 25 mm Hg) and if lymphatics are unable to decompress the resultant transudated fluid, acute pulmonary edema results.

Hemoptysis
Causes:
Sudden hemorrhage (pulmonary apoplexy) due to the rupture of thin walled and dilated bronchial veins when there is a sudden increase in left atrial pressure. This complication is rarely life-threatening, despite the large amount of blood.

Blood tinged sputum induced by severe coughing associated with paroxysmal nocturnal dyspnea or bronchitis: commonest cause

Pink frothy sputum resulting from pulmonary edema

Pulmonary infarction due to an embolism or associated with congestive heart failure

## Causes of rapid worsening of symptoms in a case of MS:

Any condition which leads to *increase in transmitral gradient* will cause increase in left atrial pressure and will lead to worsening of symptoms of MS. The transmitral gradient increases either due to increase in cardiac output or due to tachycardia (reduced diastolic interval). Increase in heart rate is common in following conditions:

Extreme exertion

Excitement

Fever: Includes acute rheumatic fever and infective endocarditis

Severe anemia

Paroxysmal tachycardia: Most common due to atrial fibrillation

Sexual intercourse

Pregnancy

Thyrotoxicosis

### MS—Clinical features

| Severity of MS | Clinical features |
| --- | --- |
| Minimal | None |
| Mild | Asymptomatic / Mild DOE |
| Moderate | DOE / PND ± Pulmonary Edema |
| Severe | Dyspnea at rest / Orthopnea / ± Pulmonary Edema |
| Critical | NYHA IV / Severe PAH / RVF / Fatigue |

*Symptoms appear only if MVA is < 2.5 sq. cm
*Symptoms at rest appear only if MVA < 1.4 sq. cm

## Signs of MS

The physical examination, especially examination of the arterial and venous pulses and the heart, is often diagnostic for mitral stenosis.

Pulse:

The arterial pulses are normal but reduced in volume due to the decreased stroke volume.

Atrial fibrillation: irregularly irregular pulse.

Mitral facies / Malar flush:

When MS is severe and cardiac output is diminished (associated pulmonary hypertension), there is vasoconstriction resulting in pinkish-purple patches on the cheeks (mitral facies; Malar flush).

Left parasternal heave—Suggestive of right ventricular hypertrophy due to pulmonary hypertension

Grading of parasternal heave

Grade I: Mild lift easily seen than felt; made out from a tangential view

Grade II: An easily palpable lift

Grade III: A prominent lift which can be suppressed with pressure from palpating hand.

Grade IV: A very prominent lift which cannot be suppressed with palpating hand.

Right heart failure: Ankle/sacral edema, hepatomegaly

Chronic right heart failure: Ascites, cardiac cirrhosis and cachexia

## Jugular Venous Pulse in Mitral Stenosis

| Feature | Findings | Mechanism / significance |
|---|---|---|
| Level | Normal or elevated | Elevated with<br>  RV failure<br>  Associated organic TS<br>  Lutembacher's syndrome |
| Waves | | |
| A wave | Normal or prominent | Prominent A wave with<br>  Severe PAH<br>  Associated organic TS<br>  Lutembacher's syndrome |
| X descent | Normal or obliterated | Obliterated with<br>  Atrial fibrillation<br>  Severe TR |
| V wave | Normal or prominent | Prominent V wave with<br>  RV failure<br>  TR |
| Y descent | Normal/Rapid/Slow | Rapid Y descent with<br>  RV failure<br>  TR<br>Slow Y descent with<br>  Associated TS |

# Auscultation in MS

**Sounds**:

Classical findings:

S1: Loud

S2:  Pulmonary component of S2 is loud due to pulmonary hypertension

S3: Absent in pure MS (except RV S3)

S4: Absent (Rarely RV S4 due to PH)

Opening Snap (OS): Present

Ejection click (EC):  Pulmonary EC may be present

S1: Loud

S1 is 'loud' if
S1 is louder than A2 at base
Palpable S1

**Loud S1:**

*Correlates with presence and intensity of OS*
*Indicates pliable leaflets*
*Rules out significant MR*
*Does not correlate with severity of MS*

**Common causes of MS with soft S1/OS**

Severe pulmonary hypertension and RVH
Calcific mitral valve
CHF or low output states
Dominant MR
Associated moderate AV disease
Mild MS

**Significant MS with normal OS and soft S1:**

MS with prolonged PR interval

**Mechanism of loud S1 in MS**

Wide open MV at end of diastole (high LAP)
MV closure at higher left ventricular pressure
Delayed MV closure
Thickened but pliable MV leaflets

**Other causes of loud S1 (other than MS)**

Exercise
Hyperkinetic circulatory states
ASD
Sinus tachycardia
Short PR interval

**S2: Loud P2; A2 normal**

*Loudness of P2 is useful in grading pulmonary hypertension*

| | |
|---|---|
| P2 = A2: | Mild PH |
| P2 > A2: | Moderate PH |
| P2 >> A2: | Severe PH |

\*    *Left parasternal heave is more specific sign of pulmonary hypertension than loud P2*

S3:
    LV S3:
        **Never** heard in pure MS
        Its presence is an excellent evidence of at least moderate MR (Mixed mitral valve disease)
        If present, BMV should not be done (as it is suggestive of significant MR)

    RV S3: May be present in MS due to RHF

    S4: Not present in MS
    RV S4 may be present due to pulmonary hypertension

\*    *Either S3 and / or S4 of left ventricular origin essentially excludes significant MS*

**Additional sounds in MS:**
1. Opening snap (OS)
2. Ejection click (EC)

    **1. Opening snap (OS):**
    Sign of dominant MS (of rheumatic origin)

    **Absent OS in a case of MS suggests**
        Associated significant MR
        Congenital MS
        Severe calcification of MV
        Severe PH (> 10 Wood units)
        Massive LA thrombus
        Associated moderate AV disease
        Severe subvalvular (of MV) crowding

## OS in absence of MS

MV origin:
>MR
>VSD
>PDA

TV origin:
>TS
>TR, Ebstein's
>ASD
>HCM

*OS may be mistaken for P2.* The following points help to differentiate between these two:

*Factors favoring OS:*
>Decreased intensity in inspiration (In absence of LBBB)
>Split widens on standing
>Split narrows in inspiration (in absence of LBBB)
>2nd component is as loud at apex as at LSB
>Loud S1
>If triple sound is present at LSB

*Differentiation between OS and S3:*

*Factors favoring OS:*
>Sharp and shorter
>Higher pitched sound
>Well heard even at left sternal edge
>Closer to A2 as compared to S3

** An ***easy way to remember the following intervals***:
>A2 to S4 gap: 0.32 sec (Range: 30-36 msec)
>A2 to S3 gap: 0.16 sec (0.14-0.18 sec; **half of A2-S4 gap**)

A2 to OS gap: 0.08 sec (0.06-0.12 sec; **half of A2-S3 gap**)
A2 to P2 split: 0.04 sec (0.02-0.06 sec; **half of A2-OS gap**)

## A2-OS Gap

Factors affecting A2-OS gap
Increased:
HT
AS
LV dysfunction
Bradycardia
Decreased:
MR
Tachycardia

## Grading of severity of MS based on A2-OS gap

| A2-OS gap | Severity of MS |
|---|---|
| < 0.08 sec | Severe |
| > 0.10 sec | Mild |

\* *A short A2-OS interval always indicates severe MS but the converse is not true*

2. **Ejection click (EC):**
Not heard in pure MS unless severe PH is present
(Pulmonary EC in a case of MS indicates severe PH)

**Murmurs in MS**

**MDM:**
Low pitch, rough diastolic rumble
Usually localized to the 'apex'; best heard with bell of
stethoscope

Best heard in left lateral position with breadth held in expiration

Length is proportional to severity whereas intensity is linked to thrill

Thrill indicates mobile cusps

Thrill of MS (diastolic) is seen in less than 20 % of patients with dominant MR and always indicates associated **organic** MS in such patients

Thrill is less than half as frequent in presence of severe PH as without severe PH

**Presystolic accentuation (PSA):**

Sign of MS but does not indicate severity

Presence is excellent evidence against associated **significant** MR

Due to

LA contraction

Mitral annular contraction

Usually absent after onset of AF

According to **some authorities**, PSA is present in AF also. According to them, ventricular contraction starts before S1 (first heart sound). This causes mitral annular contraction leading to increase in stenosis and is partly responsible for PSA. This explains the presence of PSA in AF. PSA is usually heard if LAP is more than 10 mm Hg. Hence it is usually present in AF with short R-R intervals. PSA in AF with long diastolic cycles indicates severe MS.

**Absence of PSA in MS:**

AF

Mild MS

Prolonged PR interval

Bradycardia

Elevated LVEDP

**PSM at tricuspid area**

> Indicates associated TR.

> It reflects significant pulmonary hypertension (PASP > 60 mm Hg)

**Pulmonary regurgitation (Graham Steell's) murmur**

> Indicates severe PH

> In a study of patients with severe MS and Graham Steell's murmur;

>> In about 55 % cases the PH was > 10 Wood units

>> Rest 45 % had PH of 6-9 Wood units.

## Common causes of Severe MS with short MDM

> Low flow states: Very severe MS, Severe PH, CCF, AF with fast VR

> MV: Severe Calcific MS, Severe subvalvular crowding, LA thrombus

> Associated cardiac condition: AV disease, ASD (Lutembacher's syndrome), Severe PH and RV enlargement

> Others: Obesity, COPD etc

> \* Silent MS is uncommon with coexisting significant MR

## Common causes of prominent diastolic sounds/murmurs in absence of MS

Severe MR

L → R shunts: VSD, PDA

Increased flow across TV: ASD, Ebstein's anomaly

High grade AV block

Increased flow states: Thyrotoxicosis, Anemia

## Criteria of Severe MS

Long MDM (more than 2/3rd of diastole) with PSA (with no gap between MDM and PSA)

Decreased A2-OS gap (< 0.08 sec)

Signs of severe PH and RHF

Symptoms of NYHA class IV and chronic atrial fibrillation

Old methods:

Simultaneous phonocardiography and ECG recording:

Increased (Q-S1) – (A2-OS): Well's index.

Increased (Q-S1) / (A2-OS) ratio


## Mixed Mitral Valve disease

MS with MR

### Following points indicate a dominant MR:

LV apex: Hyperdynamic and s/o LV dilatation (down and out)

S1: Soft/Normal

Absence of OS

Presence of LV S3

Loud PSM at apex with systolic thrill (Grade 4 murmur indicates more than grade 3 MR in 60 % cases)

Short MDM without PSA

# MS: Natural History

Progressive and lifelong disease
Slow and stable in the early years
Progressive acceleration in the later years
ARF to symptom onset: Western literature: 20-40 year latency
10 yrs of symptoms
before    disabling
symptoms

10-year survival

| | |
|---|---|
| Asymptomatic: | 84 % |
| Class II symptoms: | 42% |
| Class III symptoms: | 15% |
| Class IV: | 0 % |
| NSR vs. AF: | 46% vs. 25% |

Severe PAH: Mean survival:    3 years

Western Series:

Acute rheumatic fever (ARF) progresses to symptomatic mitral stenosis in 12-15 years time. Once symptomatic, the disease acceleration is fast and NYHA class III to IV symptoms develop within 3- 4 years.

**Rowe et at**

1925-1947
N = 250
Follow up of 20 yrs

| Severity at diagnosis | Same (%) | Worse (%) | Dead (%) |
|---|---|---|---|
| NYHA Class I | 24 | 14 | 62 |
| NYHA class II | 4 | 4 | 92 |
| NYHA class III | 8 | 0 | 92 |
| Overall | 13 | 8 | 79 |

**Olesen et al**

1933-1948
N = 271
Follow up of 20 yrs

| Severity at diagnosis | Survival | | Dead/Worse |
|---|---|---|---|
| | 5 yr | 10 yr | |
| NYHA class I | - | 60 % | 40 % |
| NYHA class II | - | 20 % | 80 % |
| NYHA class III | 62 % | 38 % | - |
| NYHA class IV | 15 % | - | - |

**Munoz et al**: MS and Mixed mitral valve disease
5 yr survival rate is 45 %

**Rapaport**
Unselected mixed group of patients with mitral valve disease
N = 153
5 yr survival rate was 80 % and 10 yr rate was 60 %

## Cause of mortality in a case of MS

Progressive heart failure:     60-70 %

Systemic embolism:              20-30 %

Pulmonary embolism:             10 %

Infection:                      1-5 %

# MS: Complications

Atrial arrhythmias
Systemic embolization (10-25%)
Pulmonary infarcts
Hemoptysis
Endocarditis
Pulmonary infections
Pulmonary edema
CHF / RVF

### MS: Atrial Arrhythmias

Premature atrial contractions
Paroxysmal atrial tachycardias
Atrial flutter and/or fibrillation
    AF develops in about 30% to 40% of cases
    Incidence of AF increases with
        Age           (>40 yrs: 60%)
        LA size      (>40 mm: 50%)
    The onset of atrial fibrillation is a common cause of clinical decompensation in a case of MS. With atrial fibrillation, there is loss of atrial contraction which plays an important role in the generation of adequate left atrial pressure to maintain blood flow across the stenotic valve. Atrial fibrillation has

other deleterious effects including an increase in heart rate and, due to the reduction in the duration of diastole, a decrease in the time available for filling of the left ventricle. It also predisposes to formation of thrombi.

AF indicates poor prognosis: 25 % Vs 46 % survival at 10 yrs follow up (NSR vs AF)

AF in a young patient with 'mild MS'
    Associated ASD
    Thyrotoxicosis
    Recurrent pulmonary embolism
    Sick sinus syndrome

## MS: Embolization

Predictors of embolism in patients with mitral stenosis
    Presence of left atrial thrombus (relative risk 37)
    Degree of reduction in mitral valve area (relative risk 16.9)
    Presence of significant aortic regurgitation (relative risk 22.4)
    Size of the left atrium and its appendage, and
    Presence of atrial fibrillation
    Transient atrial fibrillation and infective endocarditis should also be considered when embolization occurs in patients with mitral stenosis who are in sinus rhythm.

Most emboli originate from the left atrium. The most common site for embolism from this site is the cerebral circulation, but any organ may be involved, especially spleen, kidneys, and the coronary circulation (resulting in a myocardial infarction). Emboli can also arise from the right atrium when there is pulmonary hypertension and right ventricular and atrial dilatation. Emboli from this site lead to pulmonary embolism and infarction

Systemic embolization

        10-20% of patients with MS

        60-70 % Emboli are cerebral

        LA thrombi have been found during surgery in 15%-20% of cases

        Risk of embolization

            High risk with:

                Increasing age of patient

                    Less than 35 yrs:  9 %

                    More than 35 yrs:  24 %

                        Couldshed et al

                Presence of AF (Only 20 % cases occur with normal sinus rhythm)

                History of prior embolism

                Associated CHF

                    $1/3^{rd}$ of emboli occur within 1 month of onset of CHF

                    $2/3^{rd}$ occur within 1 year

        Risk of embolization is more than 50% in 4.5 yrs of severe MS

        High risk if age is > 35 - 40 yrs

        No simple correlation with MVA

        Mortality:  20 %

Pulmonary embolization:

        Due to thrombi from RA or peripheral veins

        Incidence:

            15-20 % per year (Compared from 4-5 % per year in non rheumatic AF)

## MS: Endocarditis

Infective endocarditis:  Since the mitral valve is deformed, there is the potential for infective endocarditis. This complication is primarily associated with **mild** mitral stenosis when the valve is stiff and fibrotic. Endocarditis is uncommon once the valve becomes calcified and very rigid.  However, pure MS is a relatively **un**common cause of IE.  IE is more common with mixed MV disease or with pure mitral regurgitation.

## Right side congestive heart failure

Chronic pulmonary hypertension eventually leads to increased right ventricular and right atrial pressures, right ventricular enlargement, tricuspid regurgitation, and signs of right sided congestive heart failure.

## Hoarseness (Ortner's syndrome)

Results from paralysis of left recurrent laryngeal nerve
Also known as Cardiovocal syndrome
Compression of the nerve occurs between enlarged and tensed **left PA** and the **aorta** at the ligamentum arteriosum.

### Other causes of Ortner's syndrome

| | |
|---|---|
| Congenital | Atrial or ventricular septal defect, Double outlet right ventricle, Eisenmenger's complex, Patent ductus arteriosus, Ebstein's anomaly, Aortopulmonary window |
| Mitral valve disorders | Mitral stenosis, regurgitation, prolapsed |
| Aortic aneurysms | Saccular, atherosclerotic, pseudoaneurysms, dissections, traumatic, mycotic |

Adult cardiovascular disorders

|  | Left atrial enlargement, left ventricular aneurysm, pulmonary hypertension, ductus aneurysm, pulmonary embolism, thrombosed giant left atrium, tortuosity of great vessels, atrial myxoma |
| Iatrogenic | Cardiac or thoracic surgery, defibrillation, atrial fibrillation ablation procedure, repair of thoracic aneurysms |
| Miscellaneous | Foreign body causing oesophago-broncho-aortic fistula |

## MS: Hemoptysis

**Causes of hemoptysis:**

Massive hemoptysis: Due to ruptured bronchial veins (present in PAH)

Blood stained sputum: Due to PND

Pink frothy: Secondary to pulmonary edema

Chronic bronchitis

Pulmonary Infarcts

# Juvenile MS

Term coined by S. Roy.

Definition:   Mitral stenosis in a patient of less than 20 yrs of age
              (Some define it less than 18 yrs of age)

Characteristics of Juvenile MS:
  The left atrium is non compliant and hence
    LA is small
    Less incidence of AF:  Since LA is small (Incidence of AF is
      higher with large LA dimension)
    Less embolic episodes:  As incidence of AF is less
  Characteristics of MV:
    Severe subvalvular crowding
    Less calcification:  As the total duration of disease is less, the
      valve has less chance to develop calcification.  These patients
      come to attention early due to high physical activities and
      non compliant LA leads to early symptoms of pulmonary
      hypertension.
  Severe PH:  Due to non compliant LA; the LAP is high leading to
    early development of PH
  Good response to BMV:  As valve is less calcific, the MV scores are
    less and hence good results with BMV.

# Investigations

## ECG in MS

Left Atrial Enlargement (LAE):

P Mitrale: > 0.12 s in lead II: With progressive LAE, the P wave is notched in inferior leads. If the distance between 2 peaks of P wave is more than 1 small square it is the **most specific sign** of LAE.

Terminal negative P force in V1 > 0.003 mVsec (practical rule: > 1 small square of ECG): **Most sensitive sign of LAE**

Macruz index: Ratio of P wave and PR segment
> 1.6: Indicates LAE
< 1.2: No LAE
1.2-1.6: Borderline cases

P wave axis between + 45 to –30° (left axis deviation compared to normal p wave axis)

Biatrial enlargement in cases of severe PH due to MS

QRS Axis
Less than + 60°: Suggests a MVA more than 1.3 sq. cm
More than + 60°: Suggests a MVA less than 1.3 sq. cm
More than + 80°: Indicates severe PH
More than + 150°: Indicates suprasystemic PH

Pulmonary hypertension on ECG

Right ventricular systolic pressure (RVSP) more than 70 mm Hg (Severe PH):

IRBBB

R/S in V1 > 1

QRS axis more than 80°

Zone of transition right to mid precordial leads

RVSP more than 100 mm Hg:

Signs of RVH on ECG are always present

AF

Coarse fibrillatory waves (> 0.1 mV in V1)

Coarse waves indicate a larger LA than in patients with fine fibrillatory waves

Related to size and extent of fibrosis of left atrial myocardium, duration of atriomegaly and age of the patient

# CXR in MS

LAE:

    Size of left atrium does not correlate with severity of obstruction

    One of the early signs on CXR

    Signs:

        Straightening of Left heart border ("Mitralization")

        **Cause of Mitralization**

            Less prominent aortic knuckle

            Obliteration of pulmonary bay due to dilated MPA and LPA

            Dilated LAA

            Straightening of convex contour of LV due to small LV in MS

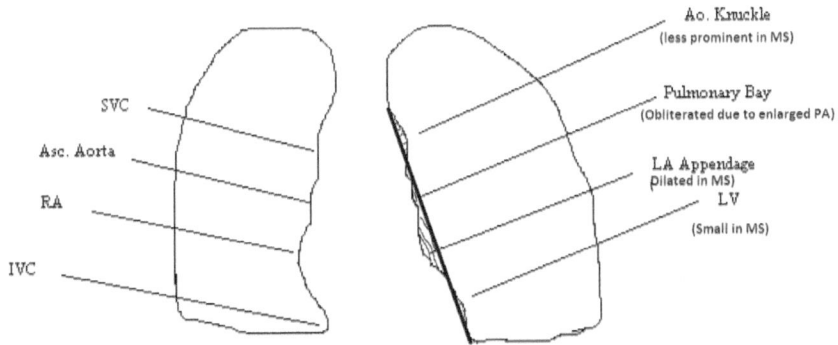

    Double density of atria

    Widening of angle of 'Carina': > 75⁰

    Compression of left bronchus and collapse of left lung

    'Sickle' shaped esophagus on Barium swallow: The most specific sign

Pulmonary venous congestion

    Prominent upper lobe veins ("Cephalization")

    Kerley B lines

    Pulmonary edema

Rarely, interlobar effusions (Kerley C lines) and in more severe cases, Kerley A lines (straight dense lines running toward the hilum) may be seen

Pulmonary arterial hypertension:

Dilated PA

Diameter of RPA at its widest point distal to the right middle lobe artery is the best estimate of pulmonary hypertension. > 20 mm is quite specific for PH

RVE

RAE

Calcification of MV

The amount of calcium present in the valve has been shown to correlate with the mean gradient across the valve.

Rarely calcific atrial thrombus can be other cause of calcification in a case of MS

# Echocardiography in MS

### Salient features:
Thick and calcific leaflets
Reduced mobility of leaflets
Commissural fusion
Subvalvular thickening and fusion
Reduction in MVA
High transmitral gradients
LAE, RAE, RVH, RVE
Associated MR, TR, PR
PAH

### Echo-MS: M Mode Features
M Mode echocardiography through the base of the stenotic mitral valve demonstrates
Increased echoes from thickened, deformed, calcified leaflets
Decreased opening amplitude of the valve
Loss of M pattern of AML and W pattern of PML: The 2 leaflets maintain a fixed relationship to each other throughout the diastole
Paradoxical motion of PML: anterior motion of the posterior leaflet
A characteristic feature but is absent in 10-17% cases
Decrease in the initial diastolic leaflet closure (EF slope).
An EF slope less than 10mm/sec indicates severe MS.
Left atrial enlargement is usually also readily apparent on M mode.
Mitral valve annular calcification can also be detected on M mode

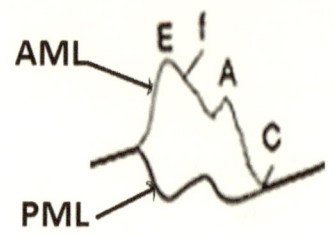

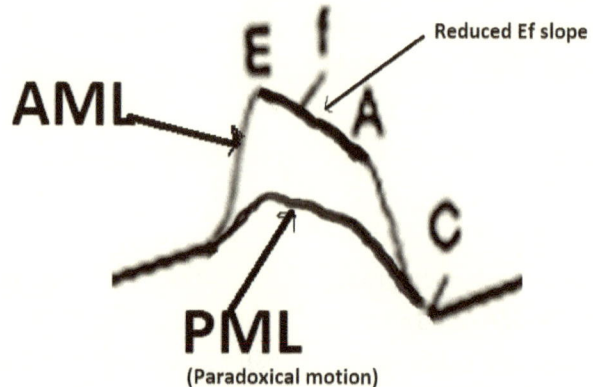

(Paradoxical motion)

Decreased EF Slope:

    Normal: > 80 mm/sec

    Other causes of reduced EF slope:

        Reduced LV compliance

        LA myxoma

        Pulmonary Hypertension

    It is not a definite marker for severity of MS

LA-AO ratio:

    Normal: $0.93 \pm 0.13$

    MS: $1.93 \pm 0.48$

## Echo-MS: 2 D Features

Hockey stick appearance of AML in diastole and immobility of PML
Doming of valve

'Fish mouth' appearance of mitral valve in PSAX and restricted opening

Thick, fibrosed and calcific valve

Subvalvular crowding

MV score (Wilkins) is based on 2 D features

Any associated complications e.g., clot, vegetation etc.

**Anatomical classification of the mitral valve (Wilkins score):** A scoring system based on 2 D echo feature in MS. Based on 4 characteristic of mitral valve (Leaflet thickening; mobility; sub valvar thickening and valvar calcification); each scored from 1-4 depending on the characteristic features as mentioned by Wilkins. A lower score (≤ 8/16) suggests more likelihood of optimal result from BMV.

| Score | Characteristics |
|---|---|
| Leaflet mobility | |
| 1 | Highly mobile valve with restriction of only leaflet tips |
| 2 | Mid portion and base of leaflets have reduced mobility |
| 3 | Valve leaflets move forward in diastole mainly at base |
| 4 | No or minimal forward motion of leaflets in diastole |
| Valvar thickening | |
| 1 | Near normal leaflets (4-5 mm) |
| 2 | Mid leaflet thickening, pronounced at margins |
| 3 | Thickening throughout leaflet (5-8mm) |
| 4 | Pronounced thickening of all leaflet tissues (> 8-10 mm) |

Sub Valvar thickening

| | |
|---|---|
| 1 | Minimal thickening of chordae just below valve |
| 2 | Thickening of chordae up to $1/3^{rd}$ of valve |
| 3 | Thickening up to distal third of valve |
| 4 | Extensive thickening and shortening up to papillary muscle |

Valvar calcification

| | |
|---|---|
| 1 | A single area of increased echo brightness |
| 2 | Scattered areas of brightness confined to margin |
| 3 | Brightness up to mid portion of leaflets |
| 4 | Extensive brightness through most of leaflets |

Total score 4 x 4 = 16

## Anatomical classification of mitral valve (Cormier et al)

Group I—Pliable non calcified AML and mild sub valvar disease (thin chordae > 10 mm long)

Group II—Pliable non calcific AML and severe sub valvar disease (thick chordae < 10 mm long)

Group III—Calcification of mitral valve of any extent

## Univ. Of South California Score

JACC; 1995: 25

Leaflet motion

| Score | Characteristics H / L ratio* |
|---|---|
| 0 (Mild) | $\geq 0.45$ |
| 1 (Moderate) | 0.26-0.44 |
| 2 (Severe) | $\leq 0.25$ |

* H / L: Height (H) and length (L) of dome of MV

Leaflet thickness

Score            Ratio of MV / PW Ao thickness**
0 (Mild)         1.5-2.0
1 (Moderate)     2.1-4.9
2 (Severe)       ≥ 5.0
** PW Ao thickness: Thickness of aortic posterior wall

Subvalvular thickening

0 (Mild)         Thin faintly visible chordae tendineae
1 (Moderate)     Areas of echo density equal to
                 endocardium
2 (Severe)       Areas denser than endocardium and
                 thickened chordae tendineae

Commissural calcification

0 (Mild)         Homogenous density of MV orifice
1 (Moderate)     Increased density of either anterior or
                 posterior commissure
2 (Severe)       Increased densities of both commissures

## Assessment of mitral valve area & severity of MS on echocardiography

### By Planimetry:

In PSAX
    Most accurate except in following conditions:
        Low output
        AF
        S/P BMV
        Calcification and extreme distortion of anatomy
            (due to increased tissue gain MVA is difficult
            to measure)
    The technique is largely operator dependent.

Proper alignment of the imaging plane relative to valve orifice is critical. Improper alignment may make the orifice appear larger or critical than it actually is.

The orifice should be measured during initial diastole when the valve is maximally distended. Selecting an orifice recorded after valve closure has begun will result in a falsely lowered mitral valve area.

Appropriate receiver gain settings are necessary to prevent over or underestimation of the orifice area.

The orifice should appear fish--mouthed. Good lateral resolution is necessary to identify the medial and lateral margins correctly.

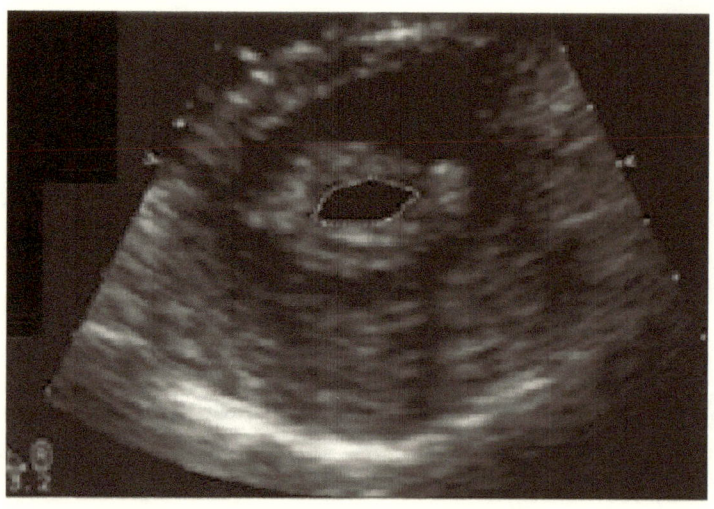

**By Pressure half time (PHT):**

Based on the concept that the rate of pressure (transmitral gradient) decrease across the stenotic MV is determined by the cross sectional area (CSA) of the orifice. The smaller the area, slower is the rate of pressure decline and less steep is the slope. Thus PHT is the time interval (in msec) between the peak early diastolic gradient and the time point where the pressure gradient is half the maximum value. During PHT measurement, dominant slope is measured; the early spike or late curvature is ignored.

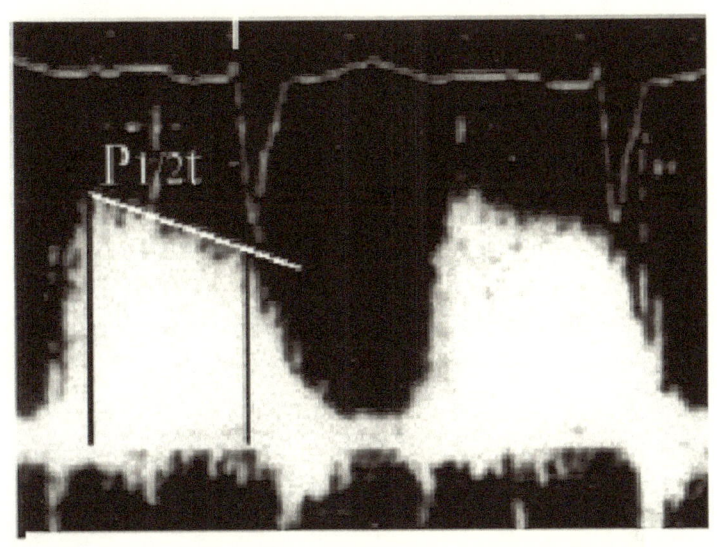

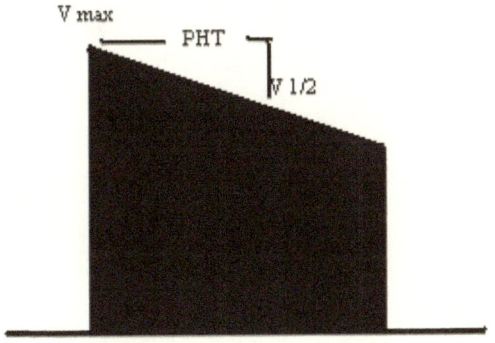

V Max: Maximal velocitty
V 1/2: Velocity at 1/2 pressure
PHT: Time interval between V max and V 1/2

The MVA is calculated by empirical formula proposed by Hatle and Angelsen

MVA = 220/PHT in msec

Inaccurate if associated with
  Reduced LV compliance
  MR
  AR
  S/P BMV (immediately after valvotomy; Due to altered atrial
    and ventricular compliance for initial 48 hrs post BMV and
    due to L → R shunt across transseptal site)

PHT is not influenced by cardiac output, duration of diastole per
beat, and it does not change during exercise.

| Values: | PHT |
| --- | --- |
| Normal: | 20-60 msec |
| Mild MS: | 90-150 msec |
| Moderate MS: | 150-220 msec |
| Severe MS: | < 220 msec |

*Patients with mitral stenosis have pressure half times of greater
than 90 msec

MS with AF: Due to beat to beat variability it is difficult to measure
MVA by PHT.
  For accurate measurements, a beat should be selected if
    Duration of selected beat is more than 300 msec
    The terminal velocity of the selected beat is more than
      1m/s
    RR interval preceding the selected beat is more than 800
      msec (suggests adequate diastolic filling period)

**By Transmitral gradient (TMG)**

In PLAX view
The TMG is calculated in mm Hg by tracing the mitral inflow ve-
locity curve
Based on Modified Bernoulli's equation

| Mean gradient (mm Hg) | Severity of MS |
|---|---|
| < 5 | Mild |
| 6-12 | Moderate |
| > 12 | Severe |

Limitations:
>Flow dependent
>Heart rate dependent
>Inaccurate if additional valvular disease (AV disease / associated
>>MR) is present

## PISA (Proximal Isovelocity Surface Area)

The proximal isovelocity surface area (PISA) or flow convergence method of calculating MVA relies on the assumption that flow accelerates radially in a series of hemispherical shells toward the vena contracta (narrowest point) of a stenotic orifice.

The first aliasing boundary (where the velocity reaches the Nyquist limit and the Doppler color changes) as flow begins to accelerate toward the stenotic mitral valve orifice is identified in the apical four chamber view.

The peak distance from the orifice to the boundary is measured at a low aliasing velocity (Va) during early diastole.

Selection of an appropriate aliasing velocity is important to prevent over or underestimation of valve area. Low aliasing velocities result in an increased distance from the flow convergence region to the stenotic valve orifice and thereby reduce measurement error (Deng et al).

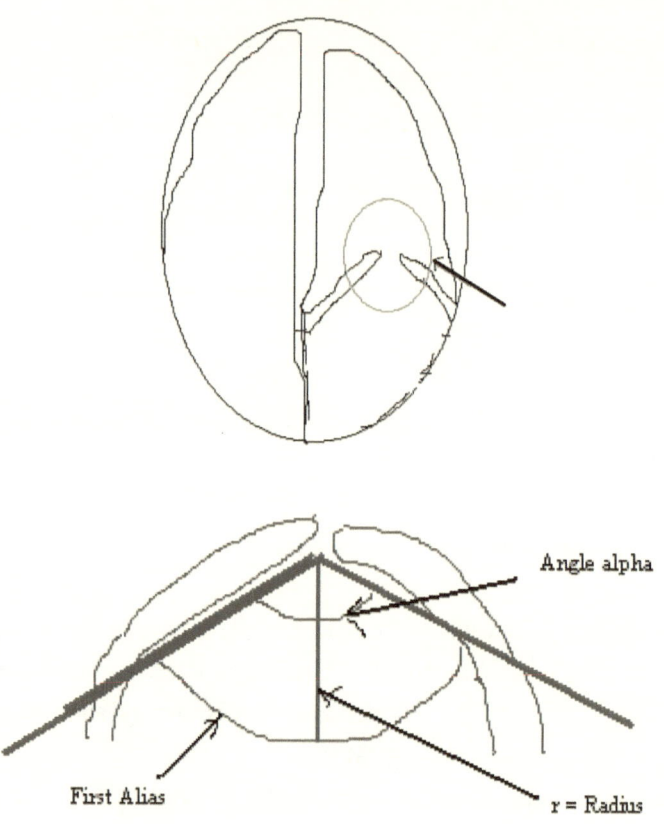

Angle alpha

First Alias

r = Radius

Calculation of MVA:

Steps

Calculate the flow

MVA is calculated with help of flow (Q) and Peak velocity across MV

Calculation of flow (Q):

The flow through the isovelocity hemisphere is equal to the surface area multiplied by the aliasing velocity (Va).

The area of the hemisphere is $2\pi r^2$ where r is the maximal radius of the PISA. The factor that accounts for the inflow funnel angle formed by the mitral leaflets is the funnel angle, α, divided by $180^0$.

The flow rate of the hemisphere is described then as

$$Q = 2\pi r^2 \times Va \times \alpha / 180^0$$

Based on the law of conservation of mass and energy, the flow through the isovelocity hemisphere must be equal to the flow through the mitral valve.

Mitral valve area is then calculated as

$$MVA = Q / Vpeak$$
$$MVA = 2\pi r^2 \times \alpha \times Va / (180^0 \times Vpeak)$$

Where Vpeak is the peak flow velocity recorded using CW Doppler.

*Deng YB et al. J Am Coll Cardiol*
*1994;24:683-689*
*Rodriguez L et al. Circulation*
*1993;88:1157*

## Continuity Equation

Based on the concept that

Flow = Mean velocity X Cross sectional area

Hence,

MVA = Flow (Transmitral Stroke volume) / TVI MS

Accurate in pure MS

Any pathology which can increase transmitral flow (e.g., coexisting MR) will overestimate area and any pathology which affects TVI will be inaccurate in measuring MVA (e.g., Coexisting AV disease)

## Flow Area:

$$MVA = \pi / 4 \times a \times b$$

Where a and b are diameters of mitral flow on color imaging measured in diametrically opposite directions in apical views (A4C and A2C)

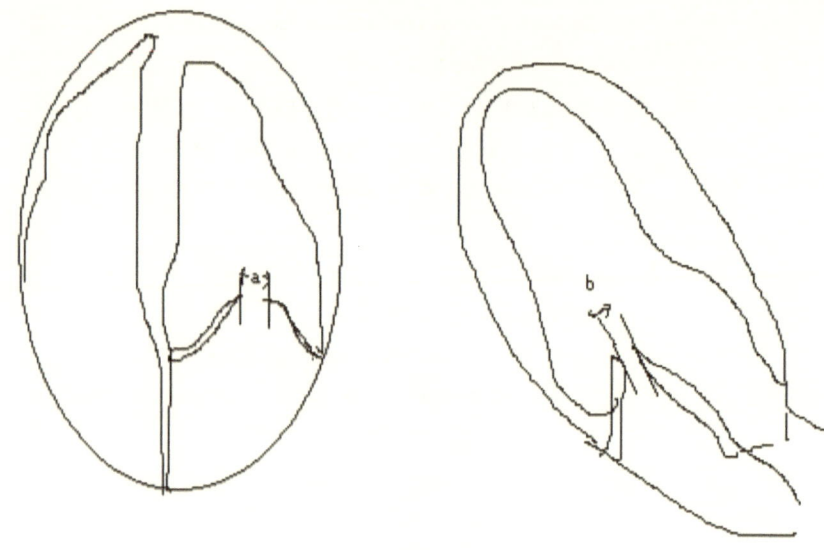

MVA by flow area
MVA = 3.14 / 4 x a x b

Not affected by coexisting MR or AR

Correlates well with planimetry area and useful if planimetry is not accurate.

### Mitral depressurization time (MDT)

Proposed by Yang and Goldberg

Similar to PHT

Based on the time taken (in msec) for the transmitral pressure gradient to fall to zero

MVA = 750 / MDT

### By Vena Contracta Width

The vena contracta is the narrowest point of flow through the stenotic mitral valve. Vena contracta width (VCW) has been recently used for evaluating mitral stenosis severity. Abaci et al measured the vena contracta width and used the following formula to calculate MVA:

$$MVA = \pi\, r^2$$
Where $r = VCW / 2$

Cardiology 2002; 98:50-59

## MS and Tissue Doppler imaging

In pure MS, Left ventricular myocardial velocities are altered as compared to healthy people. The mean LV systolic myocardial velocity, early diastolic velocity and late diastolic myocardial velocity are reduced in MS cases. However, right ventricular myocardial velocities and early and late diastolic velocities and their ratio are not altered as compared to healthy subjects. The left and right myocardial perfusion indices (MPI) can be measured and they correlate well with pulmonary hypertension in patients with pure MS.

MPI is calculated as follows:

MPI = ICT + IRT / ET

ICT: Isovolumic contraction time,
IRT: Isovolumic relaxation time, and
ET: Ejection time.

OzdemirK et al. *J Am Soc Echocardiography*2002;15:1472-1478.
OzdemirK et al. *Echocardiography*2003;20:249-256.

## Other relevant echocardiographic findings in MS:

Presence of intra cardiac clots (TEE is far superior to TTE)
Detailed morphology of MV for optimal balloon dilation (e.g., extent of calcification, any weak points in leaflets, subvalvular pathology)
Pulmonary hypertension
Associated valvular disease
LV function

# Management of MS

**Medical therapy**
Salient points:

No medical therapy will relieve fixed MS
IE and RF prophylaxis
No specific therapy in asymptomatic MS in NSR
Limitation of strenuous physical activities
In symptomatic MS: **The valve should be opened by balloon
or by surgery.** In such cases, medical therapy is indicated
till the intervention is performed.
Drug options:
**Beta Blockers (BB) or Calcium channel blockers (CCB)**
Helpful in patients with exertional symptoms
Negative chronotropic action of these drugs reduce the
extent of tachycardia due to exertion

**Salt restriction and diuretics:** If evidence of pulmonary
congestion

**Digitalis:** Indications of digoxin in MS:
AF: BB and CCB also work very well to control heart rate
Severe PH
CCF

*Medical Therapy: Atrial Fibrillation.*

Acute episode of AF with fast ventricular rate

Anticoagulation with heparin

Rate control—IV digoxin / CCB / BB

Hemodynamically unstable: DC cardioversion

Elective DC cardioversion

Warfarin for 3 weeks with INR more than 2.0

No LA thrombus on TEE

Rate control: Persistent or Permanent AF

Digoxin: effective in controlling resting tachycardia

CCB / BB: effective in controlling exercise-induced tachycardia

## Anticoagulation in MS:
## Medical Therapy: Prevention of Systemic Embolization

*Class I*

1. Anticoagulation is indicated in patients with MS and atrial fibrillation (paroxysmal, persistent, or permanent). *(Level of Evidence: B)*
2. Anticoagulation is indicated in patients with MS and a prior embolic event, even in sinus rhythm. *(Level of Evidence: B)*
3. Anticoagulation is indicated in patients with MS with left atrial thrombus. *(Level of Evidence: B)*

*Class IIb*

1. Anticoagulation may be considered for asymptomatic patients with severe MS and left atrial dimension greater than or equal to 55 mm by echocardiography.* *(Level of Evidence: B)*
2. Anticoagulation may be considered for patients with severe MS, an enlarged left atrium, and spontaneous contrast on echocardiography. *(Level of Evidence: C)*

58

**Magnitude of benefit of anticoagulation in MS**
4-15 fold reduction in events

# MS: Indication for intervention

1. Symptomatic severe MS
2. Asymptomatic severe MS
3. Moderate Mitral stenosis: Interventions should be done in following conditions even if MS is moderate:
    Symptomatic MS
    History of systemic embolism: It is said that the chance of recurrence of embolism decreases by more than 30 % if MS is relieved, even if it is not severe MS.
    If patient was symptomatic during previous pregnancy and wants to conceive again
    Surgery planned for other valves

**Recommendations for BMV for MS**

**Indications for Percutaneous Mitral Balloon Valvotomy**

*Class I*

1. Percutaneous mitral balloon valvotomy is effective for symptomatic patients (New York Heart Association [NYHA] functional class II, III, or IV), with moderate or severe MS* and valve morphology favorable for percutaneous mitral balloon valvotomy in the absence of left atrial thrombus or moderate to severe MR. *(Level of Evidence: A)*
2. Percutaneous mitral balloon valvotomy is effective for

asymptomatic patients with moderate or severe MS* and valve morphology that is favorable for percutaneous mitral balloon valvotomy who have pulmonary hypertension (pulmonary artery systolic pressure greater than 50 mm Hg at rest or greater than 60 mm Hg with exercise) in the absence of left atrial thrombus or moderate to severe MR. *(Level of Evidence: C)*

*Class IIa*

Percutaneous mitral balloon valvotomy is reasonable for patients with moderate or severe MS* who have a nonpliable calcified valve, are in NYHA functional class III–IV, and are either not candidates for surgery or are at high risk for surgery. *(Level of Evidence: C)*

*Class IIb*

1. Percutaneous mitral balloon valvotomy may be considered for asymptomatic patients with moderate or severe MS* and valve morphology favorable for percutaneous mitral balloon valvotomy who have new onset of atrial fibrillation in the absence of left atrial thrombus or moderate to severe MR. *(Level of Evidence: C)*
2. Percutaneous mitral balloon valvotomy may be considered for symptomatic patients (NYHA functional class II, III, or IV) with MV area greater than 1.5 cm² if there is evidence of hemodynamically significant MS based on pulmonary artery systolic pressure greater than 60 mm Hg, pulmonary artery wedge pressure of 25 mm Hg or more, or mean MV gradient greater than 15 mm Hg during exercise. *(Level of Evidence: C)*
3. Percutaneous mitral balloon valvotomy may be considered as an alternative to surgery for patients with moderate or severe MS who have a nonpliable calcified valve and are in NYHA class III-IV. *(Level of Evidence: C)*

1. Percutaneous mitral balloon valvotomy is not indicated for patients with mild MS. *(Level of Evidence: C)*
2. Percutaneous mitral balloon valvotomy should not be performed in patients with moderate to severe MR or left atrial thrombus. *(Level of Evidence: C)*

## Percutaneous Mitral Valvotomy

**Different techniques:**

**Balloon mitral valvotomy (BMV)**

Inoue Balloon (IB): Introduced by Inoue in 1982.

Single Balloon (SB)

Double Balloon (DB)

Multi track balloon: Bonhoeffer et al

Joseph mitral valvuloplasty (JOMIVA) balloon catheter

**Antegrade and retrograde approach to BMV**

**Metallic commissurotome (MC): Cribier's Commissurotome**

# Balloon mitral valvotomy (BMV):

Most Popular: Inoue Technique

The transseptal INOUE balloon BMV is the most popular technique

Steps

Interatrial septal puncture: Through venous access, the left atrium is entered by puncturing the interatrial septum under fluoroscopy.

MV dilatation: A stepwise dilatation of the mitral valve at the level of the commissures is performed under fluoroscopic and hemodynamic monitoring

Success has a definite initial learning curve.

Success of BMV is defined as
- a) MVA > 1.5 sq cm or ≥ 50 % increase in pre BMV MVA
- b) Immediate decrease in LA pressure < 18 mmHg (> 50% decline in transmitral gradient)
- c) Absence of any major severe complication
    - \* A decrease in pulmonary arterial pressures usually accompanies the success.

## Other Balloons used for BMV:

Single balloon (SB)

Double balloon (DB)

**Multi track balloon:** Bonhoeffer et al

Joseph mitral valvuloplasty (JOMIVA) balloon catheter

## BMV: Important points

Procedural success- About 95 %

Event free survival is more than 90% at 3-7 yrs follow up

Recommended for juvenile MS also

| | |
|---|---|
| Mortality: | < 0.5 % |
| Major complications: | < 1 % |
| Embolism, perforation | |
| MR: | |
| Severe: | 2 % |
| Mild: | 15 % |
| Residual ASD: | 10 % |

Restenosis: Defined as loss of more than 50 % of the achieved increase in MVA.

10 % (2-2.5 % per year)

## Predictors of successful BMV

Score:

Wilkins score: Total score: 16

Excellent results if total score less than or equal to 8/16

Absence of calcification of MV

Lower initial NYHA functional class

Younger Age:

46 % success at age > 65 yrs

Sinus rhythm

Atrial fibrillation: Its presence is associated with less success rate

## Contraindication for BMV

a) Left atrial thrombus

b) More than moderate MR

c) Massive or bicommisural calcification

d) Unfavorable valve morphology: High chance of tear

## Causes of MR following BMV:

Commissural

Paracommissural

Chordal rupture

Leaflet tear

Avulsion of Papillary muscle

# URGENT SURGERY Following BMV:

a) Severe MR leading to hemodynamic collapse and / or severe pulmonary edema

b) Massive intractable hemopericardium not manageable by pericardiocentesis

## Inoue Vs Double Balloon Technique

*R Arora, Khalillulah et al (JACC 1994)*

N=600

| | |
|---|---|
| Technique used: | Inoue and Double balloon |
| Age: | 27 +/- 8 yrs (Range 8-60 yrs) |
| Atrial fibrillation: | 4.3 % |
| MR ≤2: | 10.3 % |
| Densely calcific valve: | 2 % |
| Follow up: | 37 +/- 8 months (Range 6-66 months) |

Results:

Success: 98.1 % (in 2 cases; septal puncture could not be done and in 1 patient MV could not be crossed)

Optimal Commissurotomy: 93.6 %

| | |
|---|---|
| MVA (Pre) | 0.75 +/- 0.18 cm$^2$ |
| MVA (Post) | 2.2 +/- 0.38 cm$^2$ |

MR

| | |
|---|---|
| Total: | 34.6 % |
| Severe: | 1 % (Required MVR) |
| Tamponade: | 1.3 % |
| Death: | 1 % |
| Restenosis: | 1.7 % |

## Inoue Vs DB technique

Incidence of more than grade I MR was higher with Inoue technique (44 % Vs 25 %) whereas the fluoroscopic time was higher with DB technique (34 +/- 14.8 Vs 18 +/- 7 mins). No significant difference in other parameters (e.g., post procedure MVA or improvement in TMG).

**Conclusion:** BMV is safe, effective and has gratifying intermediate results. It should be considered as treatment of choice for MS

## Percutaneous transvenous mitral commissurotomy using metallic commissurotome

Percutaneous transvenous mitral commissurotomy using metallic
commissurotome: long-term follow-up results
Harikrishnan, Krishnamoorthy et al (J Invasive Cardiol.
2006 Feb; 18(2):54-8)

N = 248
64 of the procedures were for mitral restenosis after
previous valvotomy.
Success: 230 (92.7%).
TMG (mmHg)
Pre         14.54 +/- 5.79
Post        4.26 +/- 2.82 mmHg
MVA (cm$^2$)
Pre         0.85 +/- 0.12
Post        1.95 +/- 0.31
Complications

| | |
|---|---|
| Mortality | 1 (due to LV perforation) (mortality rate = 0.41%). |
| Left ventricular tear | 1 (underwent repair of the tear along with open mitral valvotomy) |

MR

| | |
|---|---|
| Severe | 4 (1 required emergency MVR) |
| Moderate | 5 |
| TIA | 1 |

Follow up

3.34 +/- 0.66 years. (6 lost to follow up)

| | |
|---|---|
| Restenosis | 7 / 224 (3 %) |
| TMG | 6.09 +/- 3.12 mmHg. |
| MVA | 1.67 +/- 0.34 cm$^2$ |

**CONCLUSION:** PTMC with metallic commissurotomy is safe and
produced good results which were sustained at a follow-up period of more than 3 years.

## Inoue Vs Double Balloon Vs Commissurotome

### Percutaneous transvenous mitral commissurotomy: immediate and long-term follow-up results

Arora et al (Catheter Cardiovasc Interv. 2002 Apr;55(4):450-6)

N = 4850
    N Db = 320 (6.6%),
    N Inoue = 4,374 (90.2%),
    N metallic valvulotome = 156 (3.2%)

Age:        27.2 +/- 11.2 years (Range 6.5-72 years)
    < 20 yrs:   1,552 (32%)

A fibrillation:   702 (14.5%)

Wilkins MV score
    ≥ 8: 1,632 (33.6%); of which 103 (2.1%) had densely calcified (Wilkins score 4) valve
    No patient was rejected on the basis of echocardiographic score using the Wilkins criteria.

Success rate:   4,838 (99.8%) patients
    Optimal result: 4,408 (90.9%)
MVA
    Pre:       0.7 +/- 0.2 cm$^2$
    Post:     1.9 +/- 0.3 cm$^2$ (P < 0.001)
    No statistically significant difference in the MVA achieved between de novo and restenosed valves
TMG:
    Pre:       29.5 +/- 7.0 mm Hg
    Post:     5.9 +/- 2.1 mm Hg (P < 0.001)
LAP
    Pre:       32.1 +/- 9.8 mm Hg
    Post:     13.1 +/- 6.2 mm Hg (P < 0.001).

Complications:

    Tamponade:        10 (0.20%)

    MR

        Appeared or worsened:    2,038 (42%)

        Severe:        68 (1.4%)

        Urgent MVR:        52 (1.1%)

Follow Up

    94 +/- 41 months (range, 12-166 months)

        MVA:        $1.7 +/- 0.3$ cm$^2$.

        Elective MVR:        34 (0.97%)

        Restenosis:        168 (4.8%)

**Conclusion:** Percutaneous transvenous mitral commissurotomy is an effective and safe procedure with gratifying results in high percentage of patients. The benefits are sustained in a majority of these patients on long-term follow-up. It should be considered as the treatment of choice in patients with rheumatic mitral stenosis of all age groups.

### Retrograde Technique of BMV:

Technique:

    Utilizes a specifically designed steerable catheter to enter the left atrium retrogradely via the left ventricle thus avoiding trans-septal puncture, an essential step in other methods of balloon mitral valvuloplasty

Retrograde non-transseptal balloon mitral valvuloplasty—an initial experience

Bahl et al (Indian Heart J. 1993 Nov-Dec; 45(6):459-62)

N = 11

Technical success:    10 (91%)

MVA (cm$^2$)

    Pre        0.8 +/- 0.2

    Post        1.8 +/- 0.4

TMG (mm Hg)
| | |
|---|---|
| Pre | 23.9 +/- 7.7 |
| Post | 8.2 +/- 2.8 |
| Major complications | 0 |

**Conclusion:** Retrograde nontransseptal balloon mitral valvuloplasty is a simple, effective and safe technique with results comparable with other techniques of mitral balloon dilatation which require transseptal catheterization. Further experience involving multi-centeric trials, is required to determine the overall efficacy of this technique for percutaneous balloon mitral valvuloplasty

**Balloon mitral valvotomy: comparison between antegrade Inoue and retrograde non-transseptal techniques (Eur Heart J 1997; Nov 18 (11); 1698-90)**
Bahl et Al

| | Antegrade BMV (n=1000) | Retrograde BMV (n=100) |
|---|---|---|
| MVA (cm $^2$) | | |
| Pre | 0.8 +/- 0.5 | 0.8 +/- 0.3 |
| Post | 2.1 +/- 0.8 | 1.9 +/- 0.8 ($p < 0.02$) |
| MR ($>/= 3$) | 1: 4% | 2: 5% ($p$ = NS) |
| Success rate | 95% | 93% |
| Complications | | |
| ASD ($> 1.5$ :1) | 2.5 % | - |
| Tamponade | 2 % | - |
| Transient LBBB | - | 28 % |
| Transient CHB | - | 2 % |
| Local | 0.5 % | 3 % ($p < 0.01$) |
| Procedure time (min) | 15 +/- 8 | 22 +/- 14 ($p < 0.05$) |
| MVA at 1 yr follow up | 1.8 +/- 0.8 | 1.9 +/- 0.9 ($p$ = NS) |

**CONCLUSIONS**: Balloon mitral valvotomy using the Inoue balloon and the retrograde non-transseptal technique results in significant immediate hemodynamic and symptomatic improvement. The Inoue technique achieved a larger immediate post-valvotomy mitral valve area, but the difference was not apparent at 1 year follow-up. Incidence of significant mitral regurgitation was similar with both the techniques; however, local complications occurred more frequently with the retrograde technique. Both techniques may complement each other in technically difficult cases.

## Mitral Regurgitation post BMV

### Natural history and predictors of moderate mitral regurgitation following balloon mitral valvuloplasty using Inoue balloon

Radhakrishnan, Shrivastava et al (Int J Cardiol. 2003 Jan;87(1):31-6)

N =                 590

Factors that predicted the development of moderate regurgitation were studied.

MR post BMV:     21 patients (3.5%) developed moderate regurgitation. They were managed conservatively.

Follow up
|  |  |  |
|---|---|---|
| At 3 months: | Mild MR: | 12 patients |
| At 1 year, | Trivial: | 5, |
|  | Mild: | 11 |
|  | Moderate: | 5. |

**CONCLUSIONS:** Patients with moderate regurgitation after mitral valvuloplasty show gradual improvement in regurgitation and symptoms. There were no factors-clinical, echocardiographic, hemodynamic or procedural factors that predicted the occurrence of moderate MR after BMV.

# JOMIVA Balloon

Evaluation of a Simplified Transseptal Mitral Valvuloplasty Technique Using Over-the-Wire Single Balloons and Complementary Femoral and Jugular Venous Approaches in 1,407 Consecutive Patients Joseph G et al. The Journal of Invasive Cardiology—Vol 17—Issue 03-Mar 2005—Pages: 132-138

Group SBT
   N = 1407
         Femoral approach:      1277
         Jugular approach:       130
Group DBT
   N = 954

Balloon used: Simple over-the-wire mitral valvuloplasty balloon catheter (Jomiva, Numed, Hopkinton, New York), by modification of a pre-existing balloon-catheter (Nucleus, Numed, inc.).

Results:

|                                    | SBT            | DBT            |
|------------------------------------|----------------|----------------|
| Optimal outcomes                   | 91.0 %         | 87.8 %         |
| Fluoroscopy time (min)             | 12.4 +/- 6.8   | 17.6 +/- 7.2   |
| Significant O2 step up (right heart) | 4.8 %        | 10.7 %         |
| Major complications rate           | 3.7 %          | 5.6 %          |
| Mean post BMV MVA (sq. cm)         | 1.92 +/- 0.31  | 2.03 +/- 0.42  |

Fluoroscopy time in jugular approach SBT-BMV ($9.0 \pm 4.2$ minutes) was significantly lower than in the femoral approach SBT-BMV ($12.4 \pm 6.8$ minutes) despite cardiac anatomic distortion.

**Conclusion:** SBT-BMV using Jomiva balloons and complementary femoral and jugular venous approaches was effective, safe, technically simple, and economical. It was comparable to and overcame several limitations of DBT-BMV.

**Technique of Jugular approach in this study.**

Right internal jugular venous and right radial arterial accesses were obtained, and pulmonary angiography was performed in a 45° right anterior oblique view to acquire a levophase image of the left atrium. Transjugular septal puncture was performed in the same view using an Endrys pediatric transseptal set (Cook). The atrial septum was punctured above the fossa ovalis about 2 cm (a vertebral body height) below the roof of the left atrium, and midway between the aorta and the anterior border of the spine. Bulging of the atrial septum toward the right facilitates obtaining a catch with the needle prior to puncture at the desired location on the septum. A 14 Fr, 20 cm long, J-shaped sheath with haemostatic valve was inserted into the left atrium, and the mitral valve was crossed using a balloon-floatation catheter. A 0.035 inch Amplatz wire with a large soft J-tip (Cook) was placed in the left ventricular apex, and valvuloplasty was performed after introducing a Jomiva balloon through the left atrial sheath.

# Management: Surgical options

## Indications for Surgery for Mitral Stenosis

*Class I*

1. MV surgery (repair if possible) is indicated in patients with symptomatic (NYHA functional class III–IV) moderate or severe MS* when 1) percutaneous mitral balloon valvotomy is unavailable, 2) percutaneous mitral balloon valvotomy is contraindicated because of left atrial thrombus despite anticoagulation or because concomitant moderate to severe MR is present, or 3) the valve morphology is not favorable for percutaneous mitral balloon valvotomy in a patient with acceptable operative risk. *(Level of Evidence: B)*

2. Symptomatic patients with moderate to severe MS* who also have moderate to severe MR should receive MV replacement, unless valve repair is possible at the time of surgery. *(Level of Evidence: C)*

*Class IIa*

MV replacement is reasonable for patients with severe MS* and severe pulmonary hypertension (pulmonary artery systolic pressure greater than 60 mm Hg) with NYHA functional class I–II symptoms who are not considered candidates for percutaneous mitral balloon valvotomy or surgical MV repair. *(Level of Evidence: C)*

*Class IIb*

MV repair may be considered for asymptomatic patients with moderate or severe MS* who have had recurrent embolic events while receiving adequate anticoagulation and who have valve morphology favorable for repair. *(Level of Evidence: C)*

*Class III*

1. MV repair for MS is not indicated for patients with mild MS. *(Level of Evidence: C)*
2. Closed commissurotomy should not be performed in patients undergoing MV repair; open commissurotomy is the preferred approach. *(Level of Evidence: C)*

**Selection of Mitral Valve Prosthesis**

*Class I*

A bioprosthesis is indicated for MV replacement in a patient who will not take warfarin, is incapable of taking warfarin, or has a clear contraindication to warfarin therapy. *(Level of Evidence: C)*

*Class IIa*

1. A mechanical prosthesis is reasonable for MV replacement in patients under 65 years of age with long-standing atrial fibrillation. *(Level of Evidence: C)*
2. A bioprosthesis is reasonable for MV replacement in patients 65 years of age or older. *(Level of Evidence: C)*
3. A bioprosthesis is reasonable for MV replacement in patients under 65 years of age in sinus rhythm who elect to receive this valve for lifestyle considerations after detailed discussions of the risks of anticoagulation versus the likelihood that a second MV replacement may be necessary in the future. *(Level of Evidence: C)*

**Operative options in mitral stenosis**

Closed mitral commissurotomy or valvotomy (CMC or CMV)
Open mitral commissurotomy or valvotomy (OMC or OMV)
Mitral valve replacement (MVR)

## Closed mitral commissurotomy or valvotomy (CMC or CMV)

First report of CMC: Cutler & Levine in 1923

Souttar performed the first successful closed mitral commissurotomy in 1925 and the technique was established by Harken and
colleagues in 1948

Incision:

5th left intercostal space (LICS)

Anterolateral thoracotomy: Usual approach

Posterolateral (it allows access through body of atrium):
Required if
Associated AF
Restenosis after previous surgical operation

Technique:

An incision is made in the left atrial appendage, followed by insertion of the right index finger into the left atrium. Initially
fingers were used for valvotomy (digital valvotomy) but since
1960, however, predominantly a Tubbs or a Dubost trans-
ventricular dilator is used. A purse string suture is placed at
the apex of the left ventricle and the dilator is subsequently
passed through the apical ventriculotomy to the mitral valve
orifice. The dilator is then positioned across the mitral valve
orifice by palpation and opened one to four times.

Dilators used: Tubbs; Dubost

Criteria of adequate valvotomy: MV should admit more than
1 and ½ fingers

## Open mitral commissurotomy or valvotomy (OMC or OMV)

Incision:

Midline sternotomy incision

Technique:

After cardioplegia, the left atrium is opened and is thoroughly
examined. Clot if present is removed. The left atrial

appendage is invaginated into the atrium and examined. Any thrombus, if present, is removed and the left atrial cavity is generously washed with ice-cold saline. Then the MV valve is examined and commissural lines are identified. The process of commissurotomy starts at anterolateral commissure. A blunt-ended, long-handled hook is placed beneath each leaflet on either side of the anterolateral commissure and carefully pulled in opposite directions. It spreads the anterolateral commissure. With a knife (no. 11 blade), an incision is made midway between valve orifice and the valve annulus. The incision should never extend to annulus; in fact, care is taken to maintain a distance of about 3 to 4 mm from the annulus. It avoids the risk of flail anterior leaflet and development of postoperative eccentric mitral regurgitation. A right-angled clamp is passed from the stab incision towards the valve orifice and is gently opened. This spreads the commissural chordae and the line of cuspal fusion is now better seen. The fused commissure between the initial stab incision and the valve orifice is incised open with a no. 11 blade or angled scissors. Then, the fused chordae are separated with knife or scissors and, if required, the incision is carried down into the center of the papillary muscle. The procedure is repeated on the posteromedial commissure. After release of fused commissural and subvalvular components, the pliability of mitral leaflets is restored by cuspal thinning. Calcification is shaved off from the leaflets and the annulus-leaflet junction. The thick fibrous layer covering the atrial surface of the leaflets is peeled off. At the completion of the procedure, some surgeons perform bilateral commissural plication. This shortens the posterior annulus and increases the coaptational area of leaflets, and thus effectively prevents any eccentric mitral regurgitation.

## Mitral valve replacement (MVR)

Risk of operation: 1% - 3%

5-year reoperation rate: 4% - 7%

5-year event free survival rate: 80% - 90%

### CMC Series: Stanley John

N= 5434;

Follow up at 15 yrs: > 70 %

Age: 27.3 +/- 9.3 yrs (6-69 yrs)

> < 20 yrs.: 25 %

Mortality: < 3 %

MR: Severe: 0.3 %; Mild: 18 %

Restenosis: 11 % at 15 yrs (4.2-11.4 per 1000 pts per yr between 5-15th yr follow up

Peak incidence of restenosis: 12 yrs

Operative mortality of restenosis: 6.7 %

> 78 % survival at 24 yrs of follow up

# Comparison of different techniques

**CMC Vs BMV**

**Important Indian series:**

**R Arora, Khalillulah et al (AHJ 1993)**
Randomized study
N = 200 (100 in each group)
Follow up:     22 +/- 6.3 months

|  | BMV (n=100) | CMC (n=100) | p value |
|---|---|---|---|
| MVA (cm$^2$) | | | |
| Pre | 0.85 +/- 0.26 | 0.79 +/- 0.21 | NS |
| Post | 2.39 +/- 0.94 | 2.2 +/- 0.85 | NS |
| MR | 14 | 12 | |
| Restenosis | 5 | 4 | |
| Death | 2 | 2 | |

**Conclusion:** Immediate and long term results with either BMV or CMC are comparable

**CMC Vs BMV (either with Single balloon [SB] or Double balloon technique [DB]): Immediate hemodynamic response to intervention**

**S Shrivastava, Sampath Kumar et al        (JTCS 1992)**

|  | CMC (n=20) | SB (n=20) | DB (n=20) |
|---|---|---|---|
| MVA (cm$^2$) | | | |
| Pre | 0.62 +/- 0.27 | 0.68 +/- 0.24 | 0.68 +/- 0.25 |
| Post | 1.5 +/- 0.5 | 1.5 +/- 0.4 | 1.9 +/- 0.8 |

PAP (mean; mm Hg)

| | | | |
|---|---|---|---|
| Pre | 49.1 +/- 17.5 | 48.8 +/- 12.3 | 46.7+/- 18.0 |
| Post | 28.6 +/- 8.3 | 34.0+/- 13.9 | 26.3 +/- 13.7 |

**Conclusion:** Single and double balloon techniques are comparable to CMC in immediate post procedure hemodynamic improvement. DB technique was associated with a larger MVA post procedure.

## B S Raju, Wynne J et al (Circ 1991)

N = 40
Follow up: 8 months

| | BMV (n=20) | CMC (n=20) |
|---|---|---|
| MVA (cm$^2$) | | |
| Pre | 1.0 +/- 0.2 | 1.0 +/- 0.4 |
| Post (1 week) | 1.6 +/- 0.6 | 1.6 +/- 0.7 |
| Post (8 mths) | 1.6 +/- 0.6 | 1.8+/- 0.6 |
| LAP (mm Hg) | | |
| Pre | 26.1+/- 4.2 | 27.6 +/- 6.2 |
| Post | 14.3+/- 7.2 | 13.7 +/- 5.4 |
| TMG (mm Hg) | | |
| Pre | 18.0 +/- 4.2 | 19.7 +/- 6.3 |
| Post | 9.6 +/- 5.1 | 9.4 +/- 4.2 |
| MR | 1 | 1 |

**Conclusion:** Results of BMC and CMC have shown comparable hemodynamic improvement and improvement is sustained through 8 months of follow up.

# BMV Vs OMV

**B S Raju, Turi Z G, Reyes et al (NEJM 1994)**

Randomized study

N = 60 (30 in each group); group matched in all aspects except gender difference

Catheterization at 1 week, 6 months and at 3 yrs of follow up

Follow Up period: 3 yrs

|  | BMV (n=30) | OMV (n=30) |
|---|---|---|
| MV score | 5-11 | 5-10 |
| PAP (mm Hg) | 23-55 | 19-64 |
| Pre procedure |  |  |
|    NYHA class II | 15 | 19 |
|    NYHA class III | 15 | 11 |
| MVA (cm$^2$) |  |  |
|    Pre | 0.9 +/- 0.3 | 0.9 +/- 0.3 |
|    Post | 2.1 +/- 0.6 | 2.0 +/- 0.6 |
|    At 3 yrs | 2.4 +/- 0.6 | 1.8 +/- 0.4 (p < 0.001) |
| Restenosis |  |  |
|    (MVA < 1.5) | 3 (10 %) | 4 (13 %) |
| Residual ASD | 4 |  |
| MR (severe) | 2 | 1 |
| NYHA class I | 72 % | 57 % |

**Conclusion:** BMV and OMV have comparable initial results with low restenosis rate. Both produce good functional capacity for at least 3 yrs. The better hemodynamic result at 3 yrs, lower cost and elimination of need of thoracotomy suggest BMV should be considered for all patients with favorable MV anatomy.

# BMV Vs CMC Vs OMV

**Farhat M B et al. Circ 1998**

Prospective randomized control trial

N = 90 (30 in each group)

MV Score: ≤ 8 / 16 in all groups

|  | BMV (n=30) | CMC (n=30) | OMV (n=30) |
|---|---|---|---|
| MVA (cm²; Gorlin Method) |  |  |  |
| Pre | 0.9 +/- 0.16 | 0.9 +/- 0.2 | 0.9 +/- 0.2 |
| Post | 2.2+/- 0.4 | 1.6 +/- 0.4 | 2.2 +/- 0.4 |
| Residual MS (< 1.5 sq. cm) | 0 % | 27 % | 0 % |

No death in any group

Follow Up data

|  | BMV | CMC | OMV |
|---|---|---|---|
| MVA (sq. cm) | 1.8 +/- 0.4 | 1.3 +/- 0.3 | 1.8 +/- 0.4 |
| Restenosis (MVA < 1.5 sq. cm) | 6.6 % | 37 % | 6.6 % |
| Residual ASD | 2 |  |  |
| MR (Grade III) | 1 |  |  |
| NYHA Class I | 87 % | 33 % | 90 % |
| Freedom from Intervention | 90 % | 50 % | 93 % |

**Discussion:**

Salient points:

1. BMV is better than CMC:

   BMV is more likely to open commissures.

   In CMC the strength is applied in two diametrically opposite direction and commissures are not in diametrically opposite direction normally.

   Larger balloons can be used if the initial inflation is not adequate in BMV.

2. Although recent studies have shown following survival rates in these 3 techniques, but due to differences in patient characteristics it is difficult to establish direct comparison among 3 techniques

   |     | 5 yrs survival rate | Event free survival |
   |-----|---------------------|---------------------|
   | BMV | 76-98 %             | 51-82 %             |
   | CMC | 90-96 %             | 72-95 %             |
   | OMV | 90-97 %             | 80-95 %             |

3. Only common drawback of BMV and CMC is, as compared to OMV there is high chance of systemic thromboembolism.

4. BMV in general is a fair risk factor for induced severe MR (> grade 3 MR in 4-6 %).

5. The restenosis rate of BMV in this series (6.6 %) is less as compared to other studies (12 % in Raju et al and other studies have shown rate up to 20 %)

**Conclusion:** In contrast to CMC, BMV and OMV produce excellent and comparable early hemodynamic improvement and are associated with decreased rate of residual stenosis, restenosis and need for reintervention. However, the good results, lower cost and elimination of drawback of thoracotomy and cardiopulmonary bypass indicate that BMV should be treatment of choice for patients with tight pliable MS.

# Choice between BMV Vs CMC / OMV: Conclusions

- BMV is better than CMC
- BMV and OMV produce excellent and comparable early hemodynamic improvement are associated with decreased rate of residual stenosis, restenosis and need for intervention.
- BMV should be treatment of choice (TOC) for suitable cases as it avoids thoracotomy and cardiopulmonary bypass (CPB): Advantage over OMV
- No need for blood transfusion and hospital stay is reduced in BMV.
- Only common drawback of BMV/CMC as compared to OMV is systemic thromboembolism

# BMV: Special Conditions

Juvenile MS
MS with pregnancy
BMV in calcific MS
Stenotic biologic prosthesis in mitral position

## Juvenile MS

### CMC: Indian series: Stanley John / G Cherian

N = 500
N = 493 (CMC done)
Success:          96.5 %
Mortality:        5.8 % (2 % in last 150 cases)
MR:
    Mild:        37.7 %
    Moderate:    7.4 %
    Severe:      1 %
Follow Up: Survival with excellent condition
    5 yr:        85 %
    10 yr:       76.8 %
Restenosis:
    3.4 % at 5 yrs follow up
    11 % in 6-10 yrs follow up

Special feature: Standard Tubbs dilators were not used. Specially constructed dilators were used for small ventricles.

## BMV in children

### Kothari et al; CCVD Apr 98

N = 45
Age: 7-12 yrs

|  | Pre | Post |
|---|---|---|
| MVA (cm$^2$) | 0.64 +/- 0.14 | 1.63 +/- 0.45 |
| TMG (mm Hg) | 24.3 +/- 7.7 | 7.9 +/- 7.9 |
| PAWP (mm Hg) | 24.3 +/- 8.6 | 14.7 +/- 7.2 |
| MR: | 3 (~ 6 %) | |
| ASD: | 2 (~ 4%) | |
| Death: | 0 | |
| Follow Up: | 20.4 +/- 16.3 months (Range 3-56 months) | |
| Restenosis: | 1 (~ 2%) | |

Special feature:
No significant difference in results if the maximum balloon size (MBS) used to dilate MV was equal to recommended balloon size (RBS) versus in group where MBS was less than RBS by 1-3 mm.

## Percutaneous transvenous mitral commissurotomy using an Inoue balloon in children with rheumatic mitral stenosis
Joseph, Balakrishnan et al
Int J Cardiol. 1997 Oct 31;62(1):19-22

| | |
|---|---|
| N (total) = | 557 |
| N (children) = | 107 |
| Age: | 14.5 +/- 2.3yrs (Range 10-18 years). |
| NYHA Class II: | 78 |
| Class III: | 29 |

All were in sinus rhythm.

MVA (cm²)
    Pre              0.73 +/- 0.18
    Post           1.7 +/- 0.53 (P < 0.001).

TMG (mmHg)
    Pre              15.6 +/- 5.2
    Post           5.1 +/- 2.3

PAP (mean; mmHg)
    Pre              41 +/- 15
    Post           28.4 +/- 10 (P < 0.001).

Complications
    Cardiac tamponade      1
    MR
        Severe           1 (required emergency MVR)
        Moderate       5 (4.7 %)
    Mortality           0
    ASD              4 (3.7%)

Follow up
    At 14 months (mean)
    MVA             1.68 +/- 0.4 cm²
    TMG             6 +/- 3.5 mmHg,
    Restenosis:       2 (1.8%)

**Conclusion:**

The immediate hemodynamic results in children were compared to 450 adult patients who underwent PTMC in the same period. The outcome was similar in both groups. Children were found to have significantly higher pulmonary artery pressure compared to adults. We found that PTMC using an Inoue balloon is very effective and safe in children, and consider that it should be the procedure of choice for young patients with symptomatic rheumatic mitral stenosis

# MS with Pregnancy

Pregnancy with severe MS:

    All eligible patients should be considered for BMV before conception.

    Those who develop class III/IV symptoms during pregnancy should undergo BMV with limited fluoroscopy and lead shielding; usually after 20 weeks of gestation.

**Balloon mitral valvotomy in pregnancy: maternal and fetal outcomes**

**(JACG 1998; 187(4); 409-15)**

Gupta, Lokhandwala et al

| | |
|---|---|
| N = | 40 |
| Age: | 24+/-5 years |
| Procedure: | BMV at 21+/-11 weeks of pregnancy. |

Special shielding was used during BMV to limit radiation to the fetus

Pregnancy was continued in 29 patients; 11 opted for MTP

| | |
|---|---|
| Success | 39 |
| MVA | |
| Pre | $0.8+/-0.2 \text{ cm}^2$ |
| Post | $1.7+/-0.2 \text{ cm}^2$ |
| Fluoroscopy time: | 7.8+/-1.9 mins |
| Obstetrics data | Full term delivery data were available in 23 babies |
| | Birth weights: 2.32+/-0.5 kg |

**CONCLUSIONS:** During pregnancy, BMV by the Inoue technique is feasible, safe, and effective. There is marked symptomatic relief, along with excellent maternal and fetal outcomes

## Balloon mitral valvuloplasty during pregnancy

(Int J Gynaecol Obstet. 2004 Apr; 85(1):18-23)

Routrav et al

| | |
|---|---|
| N = | 40 |
| Age: | 23.4 +/- 4.8 years |
| Procedure: | At 24.2 +/- 4.6 weeks of gestation |

MVA (cm$^2$)

| | |
|---|---|
| Pre | 0.82+/-0.34 |
| Post | 1.9+/-0.4 |
| Complication | 1 (pericardial tamponade) |
| Fluoroscopy time (min) | 5.5 +/- 3.8. |
| Obstetrics data: | |
| Maternal death: | 0 |
| Abortion: | 0 |
| IUGR: | 0 |
| Still birth | 1 (rest 39 babies were normal at birth) |

Follow up (of babies) Normal except 1 died due to non cardiac cause

CONCLUSIONS: During pregnancy, BMV is feasible, safe and effective. Maternal and fetal outcomes are excellent. Growth and milestone of development are not affected.

## Closed mitral valvotomy during pregnancy. A 20-year experience

Pavankumar et al (Scand J Thorac Cardiovasc Surg. 1988;22(1):11-5)

| | |
|---|---|
| N = | 126 |
| Average duration of pregnancy: | 21 weeks |
| NYHA Class ≥ 3 | 91% |
| Surgical mortality: | 0 % |
| NYHA Class (Postoperative) | 84% in NYHA class I. |

Full-term normal delivery:   82% of the pregnancies
Total fetal mortality    6%.
There were no congenital abnormalities and the infants' progress was normal

**Conclusion**: Closed mitral valvotomy during pregnancy thus was safe and reliable, giving significant functional and clinical improvement without adversely affecting the fetus.


# BMV in Calcified MS

Calcium deposits on the mitral valve are frequent and have a negative impact on BMV and surgery results.
Role of extent of calcification:

Higher the calcification score poorer is the immediate and long term success with BMV. The late event free survival rate is also significantly less with BMV

Suboptimal result in Calcific MS

Immediate success rate around 76 % (Iung et al)

High residual mitral stenosis after BMV in Calcific MS

Incidence of MR after BMV in calcific MS is **not** significantly higher than in BMV in non calcific MS

Faster restenosis rate in calcific MV

Late symptomatic deterioration is common

Only 36 ± 4% of the patients maintained good results after 8 years in one study.

Role of site of calcification

Commissural calcification is worse for outcome after BMV. If commissures are spared, BMV is likely to have good outcome.

Change of strategies

Smaller and stepwise dilatations appear to be safer

Metallic commissurotome is an alternative to BMV in Calcific MS

Surgical management (MVR or OMV) is a better option.

## BMV in calcific MS

Tajcu, Palacious et al. JACC 1994

| | Calcific MS (N=153) | Non calcific MS (N=173) |
|---|---|---|
| MVA | | |
| Post BMV | 1.8 +/- 0.06 | 2.1 +/- 0.06 |
| > 1.5 sq. cm | 65 % | 83 % (p < 0.004) |
| | | |
| Successful BMV (MVA > 1.5 sq. cm without significant MR or ASD) | | |
| | 52 % | 69 % (p < 0.001) |
| MR ≥ 2 + | 11 % | 9 % (p = NS) |
| 2 yr follow up | | |
| Survival | 80 % | 99 % (p < 0.05) |
| Survival without MVR | | |
| | 67 % | 93 % (p < 0.05) |
| Event free survival | 63 % | 88 % (p < 0.05) |

## Success rate (Of BMV) in proportion to degree of calcification

| Degree of calcification | Success rate |
|---|---|
| 1 + | 59 % |
| 2 + | 48 % |
| 3 + | 35 % |
| 4 + | 23 % |

**Conclusion:** BMV in calcific MS is not as successful as in non calcific MS

## Stenotic biologic prosthesis in mitral position.

The mechanism of stenosis on biological prosthesis is predominantly calcification and cusp fibrosis, not fusion of the commissures. Thus, BMV is unlikely to be successful in such cases. Hence, in the literature, there are sporadic descriptions of successful PMV in such situations. BMV in these cases should be restricted to highly symptomatic patients with contraindication for valve replacement

These valves are better to be replaced rather than dilated during cardiac surgery also. Lin et al. dilated the valve prosthesis in 5 patients whose valves were replaced a second time due to stenosis, and observed thereafter a lack of cusp coaptation, as well as tears on the free edges of the leaflets or along their insertion in the prosthesis ring, causing severe mitral regurgitation (MR).

# Mitral Regurgitation

# Etiology: Mitral Regurgitation (MR)

Etiology of chronic MR

Inflammatory:
RHD
Aortoarteritis
SLE
Scleroderma

Degenerative:
MV Prolapse (Myxomatous degeneration)
Mitral annular calcification
Marfan syndrome
Ehlers-Danlos syndrome
Pseudoxanthoma elasticum

Infective: Endocarditis

Structural
Papillary muscle dysfunction (CAD)
Rupture chordae tendineae (IE, CAD, Trauma, MVP, post BMV)
Mitral annular dilatation / LV dilation
HCM

Congenital

    Mitral valve clefts or fenestrations

    Parachute mitral valve

    In association with

        AV canal defect

        Endocardial fibroelastosis

        TGA

        Anomalous origin of Left coronary artery

# Rheumatic chronic MR

## Clinical Features

## Symptoms

Asymptomatic for decades

Fatigue:  Usually the initial symptom

Dyspnea on effort

      Orthopnea and PND are late symptoms (compare with MS)

**Causes of rapid progression of Dyspnea in a case of MR**

Infective endocarditis (IE)

      * MR is second only to VSD in its predilection for IE

Recurrence of rheumatic activity

Chordal rupture

Onset of atrial fibrillation

Onset or progression of coronary artery disease

Palpitations

      Atrial arrhythmias

      Increased volume overload leads to forceful contraction

      Rarely ventricular extrasystoles (more common with MR

         secondary to ischemic heart disease and MVP)

Peripheral edema:  Late and uncommon

Angina:  Uncommon

* Hemoptysis is rare in MR (compare with MS)

# Signs: Physical findings

### Pulse:
Best appreciated in carotid artery

Brisk or jerky with decreased pulse volume

Quick rising, poorly sustained and of low amplitude

Small 'water hammer' pulse

The collapsing quality becomes less marked as the severity of
MR increases and LVF supervenes

### Blood pressure
No alteration in systemic blood pressure

### Apical Impulse
Displaced and hyperdynamic

Sustained in late course

### Parasternal lift
Usually due to left atrial thrust; hence occurs late in cardiac
cycle

Rarely due to RV heave

### Jugular Venous pulse in MR

Jugular venous pressure and waveforms are usually normal in MR unless right ventricular failure develops or associated with other valvular
lesions or severe PH

| Feature | Findings | Mechanism / significance |
|---------|----------|--------------------------|
| **Level** | Normal or elevated | Elevated with<br>PAH and RV failure<br>Associated organic TV disease<br>Lutembacher syndrome |

## Waves

A wave    Normal or prominent    Prominent A wave with
                                      Severe PAH
                                      Associated organic TS

X descent    Normal or obliterated    Obliterated with
                                        Atrial fibrillation
                                        Severe TR

V wave    Normal or prominent    Prominent V wave with
                                         RV failure
                                        TR

Y descent    Normal/Rapid/Slow    Rapid Y descent with
                                        RV failure
                                        TR
                                        Slow Y descent with
                                        Associated TS

## Auscultation

### Sounds

- **S1**: Soft or normal; Muffled with murmur
  *Mechanism of Soft S1 in MR*
       Loss of isovolumic systole
       Failure of leaflets to close
       Fibrosis, shortening and diminished mobility of valve
       Myocardial dysfunction in secondary MR
  *S1: Loud or normal S1 in MR*
       Associated MS
       Rheumatic MR with well preserved AML
       MR due to MVP

**Soft S1 out of proportion to severity of MR**, i.e., Soft
S1 with mild MR
Non rheumatic MR
MR secondary to CAD and cardiomyopathies
Associated severe AR

- **S2:**
Wide split (suggests grade 3 MR); A2 normal; P2 loud
if PH develops
Wide and fixed split if associated with ASD or AV canal
defect

- **S3:** Usually present; almost always with ≥ grade 2 MR
Indicates at least moderate MR
Rules out significant MS

- **S4:** Absent in chronic rheumatic MR
Reasons:
Dilated compliant LV
Associated MS or AF
Dilated, diseased LA incapable of generating
enough force to produce S4
However, S4 is commonly present in acute MR
S4 may be present in non rheumatic MR (e.g., with CAD,
HOCM or endomyocardial fibrosis)

- **Systolic click:** MVP with MR
- **OS:** may be present

**MR: Murmurs**

- **Pansystolic murmur (PSM):**
Holosystolic (extends beyond A2)
High pitch, soft, blowing in character
Thrill indicates severe MR

* Ischemic MR murmur is rarely more than grade 3 even if severe

No change with respiration (D/D with TR)

May have late systolic accentuation

Only late systolic murmur: MR is usually mild and secondary to MVP or papillary muscle dysfunction (PMD)

Radiation

Axilla: Due to AML involvement

Sternum: Due to PML involvement

Aortic root: MR jet strikes LA wall near aortic root

Associated conditions that may decrease the intensity of PSM of MR

CCF

LV dysfunction

Low cardiac output states

Associated MS

Huge LA

Large RV

Obesity and large breasts

COPD

**MR: PSM**

**Decrease:**

Standing         (d/d MVP/HOCM)

Strain phase of Valsalva

Amyl nitrate

Exercise

**Increase:**

Isometric hand grip (d/d HOCM/AS/MVP)

Release phase of Valsalva

Squatting

* *No change with respiration and cycle length (beat to beat*

*variation):   Distinctly different from murmurs of AS and MVP with MR*

● **MDM at apex:**
   Flow murmur across MV due to significant MR.
   Never without S3 if it is due to flow murmur
   PSA is absent if due to flow murmur
   Associated with organic MS

● **PSM at tricuspid area due to TR:**
   Rare

**Criteria for Severe MR**

Symptomatic MR
Carotid pulse: Small volume and quick rising
Dilated LV with hyperdynamic quality
LA rock:  Important feature with multivalvular involvement; absent if MS is present
Presence of S3 and flow related MDM
Grade ≥ 4 PSM (Presence of thrill indicates severe MR): Controversial criteria
   *Paul Wood:  Severe MR was present in more than 58 % cases if the grade of murmur was > than 3*
   *Braunwald: There is little correlation between intensity of systolic murmur and the severity of MR*

*Characteristics of papillary muscle dysfunction (PMD)*

Precordial motion abnormalities commonly associated with papillary muscle dysfunction (PMD)
   LV heave
   Bifid or double LV apical impulse
   Cardiomegaly

Palpable S4/S3

Palpable parasternal lift

Murmur in PMD

Classic murmur has onset in early to mid systole with sound vibration extending up to S2.  S3 and S4 are common. The absence of S4 in the setting of a late systolic murmur points that murmur is not due to PMD

# Hemodynamics of MR

LA pressure
    Large V wave
    'V' wave more than 10 mm Hg than PAWP
        If 'V' wave more than 3 times PAWP it indicates significant
           MR

LVEDP
    Much lower than mean LAP or PAWP
    MR ≤ grade 3: LVEDP is normal or slightly high
    Grade 4 MR: Raised LVEDP
    MR due to CAD or Cardiomyopathy: Raised LVEDP

# Chronic Mitral Regurgitation

**Investigations**

## ECG

Left atrial enlargement:
    Biatrial enlargement if evidence of significant PH
Normal frontal plane QRS axis
Atrial fibrillation
LVH due to diastolic overload
    Tall R in left precordial leads
    S wave in V1 is small in magnitude (compare from
        other causes of diastolic overload)

## CXR

Enlarged LV
Enlarged LA
    Double density
    Widening of carinal angle
Large LA appendage ONLY occurs in *significant MR of
    RHEUMATIC origin*
Evidence of pulmonary venous hypertension
Calcification of MV
    More common with rheumatic MR

## Echocardiography

**Importance of Echo-Doppler examination in MR Helps in
    deciding**
Severity of MR
Etiology and pathophysiology of MR
Effects of MR on cardiac chambers
LVEF

Estimates PA pressure: Pulmonary hypertension
Determines prognosis
Diagnosis of associated pathology
Decision regarding type of surgery
Serial follow up.

**M Mode:**
Increased LV dimensions (LVIDS and LVIDD)
Increased LA size
Etiology of MR: Rheumatic (PML motion is restricted) versus MV prolapse (Systolic sagging of PML)
M mode of PV to diagnose pulmonary hypertension

**2 D Echo**
*Morphology/Etiology of MV disease*
Rheumatic affection:
Thickened leaflets, mild doming, restricted motion of PML and subvalvular crowding
MV prolapse:
Thin or thick (myxomatous degeneration) leaflets with evidence of prolapse during systole, redundant leaflets, incomplete coaptation, normal PML motion and usually normal subvalvular status.

*Decision about Type of surgery*
Conditions favoring **MVR**
Calcification of leaflets or annulus
Anterior leaflet involvement
Rheumatic disease
Conditions favoring MV **repair**
No calcification
Posterior leaflet involvement
Nonrheumatic disease
Ruptured chordae tendineae
Types of MV repair

Annuloplasty
Annular dilatation with short leaflets
Others like chordal shortening or lengthening, papillary muscle translocation or PML wedge resec-
tion can be decided on 2 D echo

*LVEF*

LVEF in MR with normal LV function is usually above 60 %.
For better post operative survival and LV function, sur-
gery should be timed in asymptomatic chronic MR with
LVEF of 60% and LV ESD of 45 mm.

**Severe MR: 2D signs**

Dilated LA
Dilated LV
Exaggerated systolic expansion of LA
IAS bulges from left to right
No spontaneous echo contrast in LA but present in aorta: suggestive
of severe decrease in forward stroke volume

**Spectral Doppler:**
**CW Doppler:** A4C view is used
Echo density of MR trace
Denser the signal more is the spectral broadening and
more severe is the MR
Shape of MR trace
Holosystolic jet is suggestive of classical MR
Early systolic peaking and decrescendo in late systole
with dense signals suggestive of severe MR
Early systolic peak with faint signals seen in milder MR
Estimation of LAP:
LAP = SBP – Peak gradient of MR trace
Peak gradient of MR = 4 X (V max of MR)$^2$
Sensitive test of LAP measurement in absence of

LVOTO

**PW Doppler**:

Evidence of systolic flow reversal in pulmonary veins correlates with high LAP and prominent V wave in LAP: Good criteria of severe MR

**Color Doppler study**:

Most important in assessment in MR

*Severe MR: Characteristics of 'Jet'*

Wall hugging jets

Jets entering LA appendage

Jets entering pulmonary vein or veins

Encircles the left atrium

Agitated flow seen in LA

**MR Jet area:**

Jet area:  Measured in PLAX

Grading of MR based on 'Jet' area

*Absolute jet area*

| | |
|---|---|
| Mild: | < 4 sq. cm |
| Moderate: | 4-8 sq. cm |
| Severe: | > 8 sq. cm |

*On TEE*

| | |
|---|---|
| Mild: | < 3 sq. cm |
| Moderate: | 3-6 sq. cm |
| Severe: | > 6 sq. cm |

*Jet area/LA area (Gatewood and Nanda)*

Grading of MR:

| | |
|---|---|
| Mild: | <20 % |
| Moderate: | 20-40% |
| Severe: | >40 % |

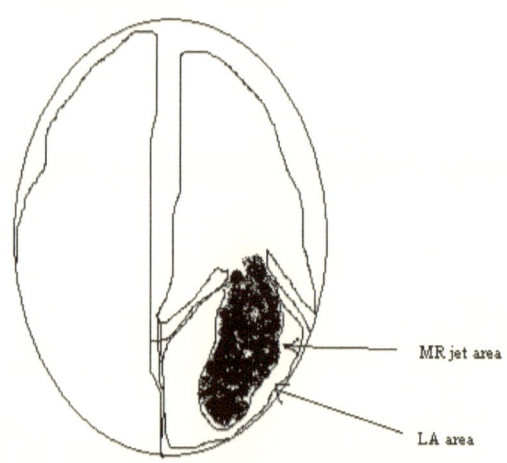

MR jet area

LA area

Criteria for Severe MR
Absolute MR jet area > 8 cm2
MR jet area / LA area > 40 %
It should be measured in all views i.e., PLAX,
Apical 4 chamber and apical 2 chamber view

*Jet width & height:  Severe MR is indicated if*

| | |
|---|---|
| Jet width (PSAX): | > 2.25 cm |
| Jet area (PSAX): | > 1.2 sq. cm |
| Jet height (PLAX): | > 10mm |

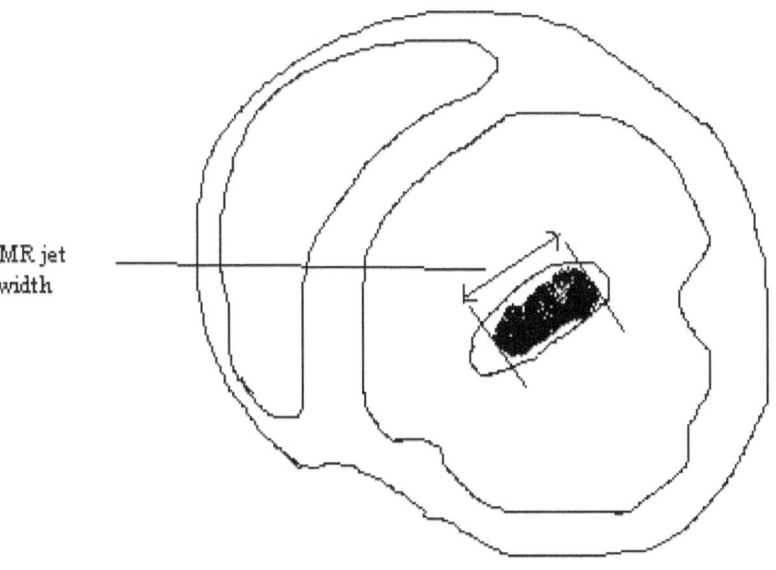

MR jet
width

Criteria for severe MR
By jet width = > 2.25 cm
By MR jet area = > 1.25 sq. cm

**Limitations of grading of MR based on jet area:**

Not accurate in eccentric MR:  Underestimates in wall hugging jets and overestimates in wall hitting jets of MR

Dependant on color gain settings

Not useful in acute MR

**Other methods to assess MR severity:**

Regurgitant Volume (RV)

Volume of blood that leaks back into LA during each systole

Effective Stroke volume = Total Mitral stroke volume (TMSV) – Regurgitant volume (RV)

Effective stroke volume = Aortic stroke volume (ASV) in pure MR

**So, RV = TMSV – ASV**


*TMSV calculation:*

TMSV= VTI MV x MV annulus area

Where VTI MV : Velocity time integral of diastolic MV flow

Other method:

TMSV = LVEDV – LVESV

Where LVEDV:  Left ventricular end diastolic volume LVESV:  Left ventricular end systolic volume

LVEDV and LVESV are measured by modified Simpson's method


*ASV calculation:*

ASV = VTI AV X LVOT Area

Where VTI AV; Velocity time integral across AV

LVOT area:  Calculated from LVOT diameter measured in PLAX view


Grading of MR on RV:

| | |
|---|---|
| Mild: | Less than 30 ml |
| Moderate: | 30-45 ml |
| Grade 3 MR: | 45-60 ml |
| Grade 4: | More than 60 ml |

**PISA method:**

**PISA stands for Proximal Isovelocity Surface Area**

The technique is based on continuity equation. Velocity of blood increases when it flows through a narrow orifice. The increase in velocity is gradual and increases as the flow approaches the orifice. It produces an area of accelerated flow near the orifice. This is seen on color Doppler as proximal turbulence converging on to the orifice, hence called as flow convergence.

The concept of PISA is that at a hemisphere placed at equidistant points proximal to the orifice, the velocity of blood flow is equal. On color Doppler halos are seen proximal to the orifice, which become more marked when the Nyquist limit (velocity scale) is reduced. The distance of halo, which shows color change from blue to red, is measured from tip of the valve. The area of the hemisphere can be calculated by the following formula:

PISA $= 2\,\pi\,r^2$ where r = distance of the halo

The velocity at the halo, which shows change from blue to red, is the aliasing velocity and equals Nyquist limit. The regurgitant volume (RV) would be calculated as:

Regurgitant volume (RV) = PISA X Velocity (Nyquist limit)

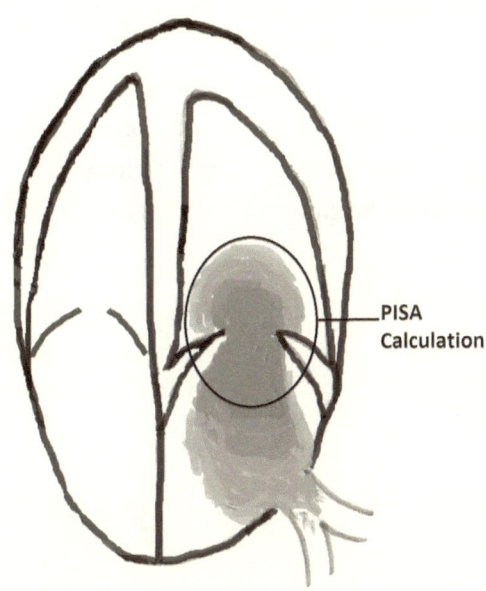

PISA Calculation

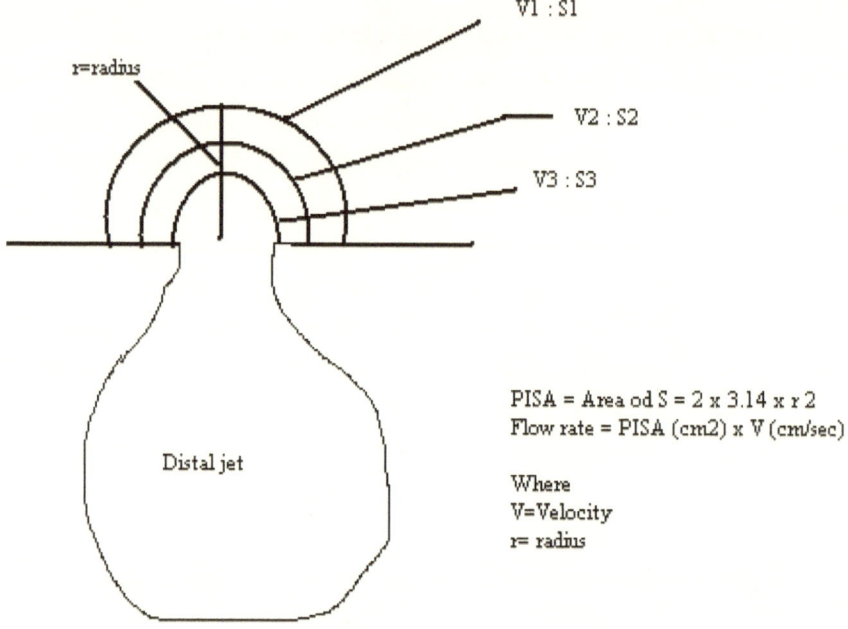

r=radius

V1 : S1

V2 : S2

V3 : S3

Distal jet

PISA = Area od S = 2 x 3.14 x r 2
Flow rate = PISA (cm2) x V (cm/sec)

Where
V=Velocity
r= radius

**Regurgitant fraction (RF):**

RF is the regurgitant volume as a percentage of total stroke volume.

RF =  RV / TMSV X 100

   =  (TMSV – FSV) / TMSV X 100

     Where TMSV = Total mitral stroke volume

             FSV = Forward stroke volume (Equal to ASV)

     (Refer to Regurgitant volume section for calculation)

**Grading of MR on RF:**

   Mild:            Less than 30 %

   Moderate:        30-55 %

   Severe MR:       More than 55 %

**Effective regurgitant orifice area (ERO):**

ERO = RV / VTI MR

Where VTI MR = Velocity time integral of MR calculated in A4C

**Grading of MR on ERO:**

| | |
|---|---|
| Mild: | Less than 0.3 cm$^2$ |
| Moderate: | 0.3-0.4 cm$^2$ |
| Severe MR: | More than 0.4 cm$^2$ |

**Vena Contracta:**

Based on the diameter of jet at its origin. As the flow pattern is not taken into account, this measurement is independent of loading conditions, independent of jet characteristics, requires no calculations and has strong correlation with severity of MR.

Vena contracta is the narrowest point of the jet where the jet seems to converge and then expand. A vena contracta of more than 6.5 mm suggest severe MR. TEE is more accurate than TTE for measurement of vena contracta.

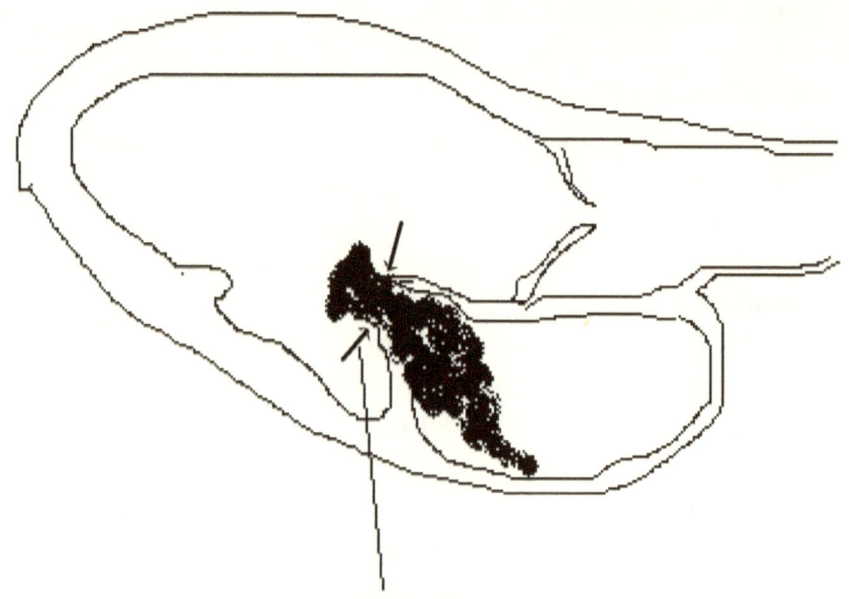

Narrowest diameter of MR jet: Vena contract

## Severity of Mitral Regurgitation by Echocardiography

- **Definite**
    - ERO ≥ 0.40 cm2
    - Regurgitant volume ≥ 60 cc
    - Regurgitant fraction ≥ 55%
    - Pulmonary vein systolic flow reversal
    - MR color flow jet reaching posterior wall of LA
    - Vena contracta width > 6.5 mm
    - 2D evidence of disruption of MV apparatus
- **Suggestive**
    - Color flow area ≥ 40% of LA size
    - Eccentric MR jet reaching posterior wall of LA
    - Dense continuous wave Doppler signal
    - Increased E velocity (≥1.5 m/sec)
    - LV dimension ≥ 7 cm
    - LA size ≥ 5.5 cm

# Cardiac catheterization

**Cardiac catheterization** is performed only if there is reasonable suspicion of CAD (or in patients more than 40 yrs of age to rule out CAD) or a discrepancy between clinical and non invasive evaluation

Angiographic grading of MR from contrast left ventriculography

| Grading | Criteria |
|---|---|
| 1 + (Minimal) | Regurgitant jet with slight opacification of left atrium and rapid clearing of contrast from left atrium. |
| 2 + (mild) | Regurgitant jet with moderate opacification of left atrium and rapid clearing of contrast from left atrium. |
| 3 + (moderate) | Marked opacification of left atrium, as dense as LV and aorta; slow clearing of contrast from markedly enlarged LA. |
| 4 + (severe) | LA more densely opacified than LV, with swirling of contrast around LA; LA remains densely opacified through complete angiography. |

# Natural History

MR tends to progress more rapidly in patients with connective tissue disease than chronic rheumatic disease.

Isolated severe MR secondary to acute rheumatic fever occurs more commonly in adolescents in developing countries and its course is rapidly progressive

Mild MR
    Stable for many years
    Only a small percentage develops severe MR

Symptomatic severe MR:  Rapaport et al
    Survival after diagnosis
        5 yrs:          80 %
        10 yrs:         60 %
    Among patients of MR on medical management, AV O2 difference and LVEDV were significant inverse predictors of survival (Cohen, Braunwald et al)

MS with MR (Rheumatic mixed mitral valve disease)
    Natural history is worse
    Survival rate
        5 yrs           67 %
        10 yrs          30 %

Other Studies
P Wood
N = 82
Mild to moderately symptomatic patients with either pure or
predominant MR
Secondary to Rheumatic fever
Concomitant MS was present in 32 out of 82 patients
Annual risk of severe disability in this series: 19 %

Ramnathen et al
N = 76; MR of diverse etiology
Symptoms
NYHA class I:        15
NYHA class II:       26
LVEF < 40 %:        20
Follow up for 4 yrs
Of 41 patients in class I/II; 9 died and 8 had ≥ class 3
symptoms
Rate of progression: 10 % per yr

Rosen et al (AJC 1994)
N=31
Asymptomatic or minimally symptomatic MR (severe) due to
MVP and normal LV / RV function
Progress to require surgical intervention: 10.3 %
Progression in patients with RV dysfunction with exercise: 14.7 %
Progression in patients without RV dysfunction with exercise:
4.9 %
Conclusion: Symptomatic deterioration is best predicted by RV
performance.

# Management of Chronic MR

- Most patients with chronic mild to moderate MR unlikely to ever need surgery
- Management is directed at
    Identifying cause and severity
    Treating underlying conditions
    Preventing complications
- Evaluating risk factors for coronary artery disease

**Management of Chronic MR: Frequency of Echocardiographic follow up**
(NEJM Vol 345, No 10, Sept 6, 2001)

| Severity of MR | LV Function | Frequency of Echo |
|---|---|---|
| Mild | Normal ESD and EF | Every 5 yrs |
| Moderate | Normal ESD and EF | Every 1-2 yrs |
| Moderate | ESD > 40 mm or EF < 65 | Annually |
| Severe | Normal ESD and EF | Annually |
| Severe | ESD > 40 mm or EF < 65 | Every 6 months |

# Medical Therapy in MR

- No generally accepted treatment in asymptomatic patients
- No long term studies suggesting benefit of afterload reduction in absence of hypertension
- ACE inhibitors if MR is associated with hypertension
- AF requires rate control, anticoagulation and at least one attempt at restoration of sinus rhythm
- No known medical therapies directly affect the disease process in the valve leaflets with MVP or rheumatic valve disease
- Acute MR
    - Diuretics :      To decrease LV filling pressure
    - Vasodilators :  To increase forward flow
                            To decrease regurgitant volume
    - Intraaortic balloon pump: To decrease afterload and to increase aortic diastolic pressure

- Chronic MR
    - Very little data on effects of medical management

## Medical Therapy for Chronic MR: Vasodilators

- Reasons for use of vasodilators
    - To decrease afterload
    - To improve aortic flow
- Data supporting use of vasodilators
    - Approximately 50 reported patients with chronic asymptomatic MR found no consistent beneficial response
    - Small group of symptomatic patients on ACE-Inhibitors, show
        - Symptomatic improvement
        - Reduction in LV size
        (Prog Card Dis, Vol 43, 6:457-475, 2001)

- Reasons to avoid vasodilators in asymptomatic patients with normal LV function
  — Afterload is usually normal
  — Unknown effects of chronic subnormal afterload
  — May mask symptoms and delay surgery

### Medical Treatment of chronic severe MR:  Results
### (NEJM 1996; 335:1417-23)

Salient points:

- Yearly mortality
  — On Medical management : 6.3%
- Morbidity at 10 yrs
  — Development of CHF : 63%
  — Chronic AF : 30%
- Baseline predictors of death
  — Higher Age, higher NYHA class, reduced EF
- Death or surgery is unavoidable within 10yrs of the diagnosis
- Surgical correction greatly improved long term survival

### Medical management: Conclusions

There is no generally accepted medical therapy which may forestall surgery for asymptomatic chronic MR.

Vasodilators (Nifedepine, ACE inhibitors) may be used in asymptomatic moderate chronic MR while on follow up.

# Indications for Mitral Valve Operation

*Class I*

1. MV surgery is recommended for the symptomatic patient with acute severe MR.* *(Level of Evidence: B)*
2. MV surgery is beneficial for patients with chronic severe MR* and NYHA functional class II, III, or IV symptoms in the absence of severe LV dysfunction (severe LV dysfunction is defined as ejection fraction less than 0.30) and/or end-systolic dimension greater than 55 mm. *(Level of Evidence: B)*
3. MV surgery is beneficial for asymptomatic patients with chronic severe MR* and mild to moderate LV dysfunction, ejection fraction 0.30 to 0.60, and/or end-systolic dimension greater than or equal to 40 mm. *(Level of Evidence: B)*
4. MV repair is recommended over MV replacement in the majority of patients with severe chronic MR* who require surgery, and patients should be referred to surgical centers experienced in MV repair. *(Level of Evidence: C)*

*Class IIa*

1. MV repair is reasonable in experienced surgical centers for asymptomatic patients with chronic severe MR* with preserved LV function (ejection fraction greater than 0.60 and end-systolic dimension less than 40 mm) in whom the likelihood of successful repair without residual MR is greater than 90%. *(Level of Evidence: B)*
2. MV surgery is reasonable for asymptomatic patients with chronic severe MR,* preserved LV function, and new onset of atrial fibrillation. *(Level of Evidence: C)*
3. MV surgery is reasonable for asymptomatic patients with chronic severe MR,* preserved LV function, and pulmonary hypertension (pulmonary artery systolic pressure greater than

50 mm Hg at rest or greater than 60 mm Hg with exercise). *(Level of Evidence: C)*

4. MV surgery is reasonable for patients with chronic severe MR* due to a primary abnormality of the mitral apparatus and NYHA functional class III–IV symptoms and severe LV dysfunction (ejection fraction less than 0.30 and/or end-systolic dimension greater than 55 mm) in whom MV repair is highly likely. *(Level of Evidence: C)*

*Class IIb*

1. MV repair may be considered for patients with chronic severe secondary MR* due to severe LV dysfunction (ejection fraction less than 0.30) who have persistent NYHA functional class III-IV symptoms despite optimal therapy for heart failure, including biventricular pacing. *(Level of Evidence: C)*

*Class III*

1. MV surgery is not indicated for asymptomatic patients with MR and preserved LV function (ejection fraction greater than 0.60 and end-systolic dimension less than 40 mm) in whom significant doubt about the feasibility of repair exists. *(Level of Evidence: C)*

2. Isolated MV surgery is not indicated for patients with mild or moderate MR. *(Level of Evidence: C)*

**Special conditions:**

**MR with pregnancy**

Usually well tolerated and rarely needs surgical intervention during pregnancy.

Vasodilators should be used only with concomitant hypertension

# Isolated Chronic Severe MR

## Chronic severe MR: Time to Intervene
*(William Stewart; JACC 1994; 24: 1544)*

Isolated Chronic Severe MR

Assess on following 5 factors:

- Symptoms
- LV size
- LV function
- Significant PH (PASP > 50 mmHg)
- Chronic or recurrent atrial fibrillation

**If ≥ 2 are abnormal:  Elective Surgery**

## Timing of Surgery
(JACC 1998; Vol 32, No 5:1486-588)

- Symptomatic patients with normal LV function
  - Normal LV function : EF >60%, ESD ≥ 45 mm
  - Patients with even mild symptoms of CHF despite normal LV function require surgery
- Symptomatic or asymptomatic with LV dysfunction
  - LV dysfunction : EF ≤ 60%, ESD ≥ 45 mm
  - Patients with LV dysfunction require surgery
    - Prevents further deterioration and improves longevity
  - Consider surgery with severe LV dysfunction if
    - MV repair is likely or
    - EF is > 30%

**Indication for Surgery:** JACC 1998; Vol 32, No 5:1486-588

- Symptomatic severe MR
- Asymptomatic severe MR if:
    — LV dysfunction at rest: < 60 % (FS < 30 %)
    — Normal LV function with
        - LVIDS:        > 45 mm or 26 mm/m2
        - LVIDD:        > 40 mm/ m2
        - LVESVI:       > 55 ml/ m2
        - LVEDVI:       > 220 ml/ m2
- Type of surgery
    — Mitral valve repair
    — MVR with preservation of mitral apparatus
    — MVR with removal of mitral apparatus
- Mitral valve repair is operation of choice
    — Preserves native valve
        - Eliminates need for anticoagulation
        - Eliminates deterioration of tissue valves
    — Preservation of mitral apparatus
        - Reduces postoperative LV dysfunction

**Types of MV surgery**

MV Repair
> MV repair requires more expertise but avoids prosthesis, anti-coagulation and risk of prosthetic valve failure.
>
> It is difficult in valve calcification, rheumatic involvement and anterior leaflet involvement but has improved post operative LV function.

MV Replacement (MVR)

> *MVR with preserved chordal apparatus ensures*
> *(As compared to MVR where MV apparatus is destroyed)*

Better post operative MV competence,
Preserves LV function and
Enhances post operative survival

Feasibility of Repair vs. Replacement (JACC 1998; Vol 32, No 5:1486-588)

- Conditions favoring repair
  - No calcification
  - Posterior leaflet involvement
  - Non rheumatic disease
  - Ruptured chordae tendineae
- Conditions favoring MVR
  - Calcification of leaflets or annulus
  - Anterior leaflet involvement
  - Rheumatic disease
- Operative Mortality
  - Repair : 2.6%
  - Replacement : 10.3%

## MR: Post operative study

**Echocardiographic predictors of LV function after correction of MR: Results and clinical implications**
Enriquez Sarano et al (JACC 1994)
- N = 266
- F/U: 8 yrs
- Post op LV function (on Echo) and 8 yr survival rate

| Post op LV function | 8 yr survival |
| --- | --- |
| < 50 % | 38 +/- 9 % |
| > 50 % | 69 +/- 8 % |

Pre op echocardiographic parameters predicting post op LV function

Univariate predictors:
Pre op LV function
Systolic diameter
Diameter / thickness ratio (LV)
End systolic wall stress
First 2 factors are multivariate predictors also

Predicted post op LVEF
= (0.45 x Pre op LVEF) – (0.48 x systolic dimension) + 42

This study suggested that if LVEF is $\geq$ 60 % and if systolic dimension is approaching 45 mm; mitral valve surgery should be strongly considered

# Summary of management of chronic severe MR

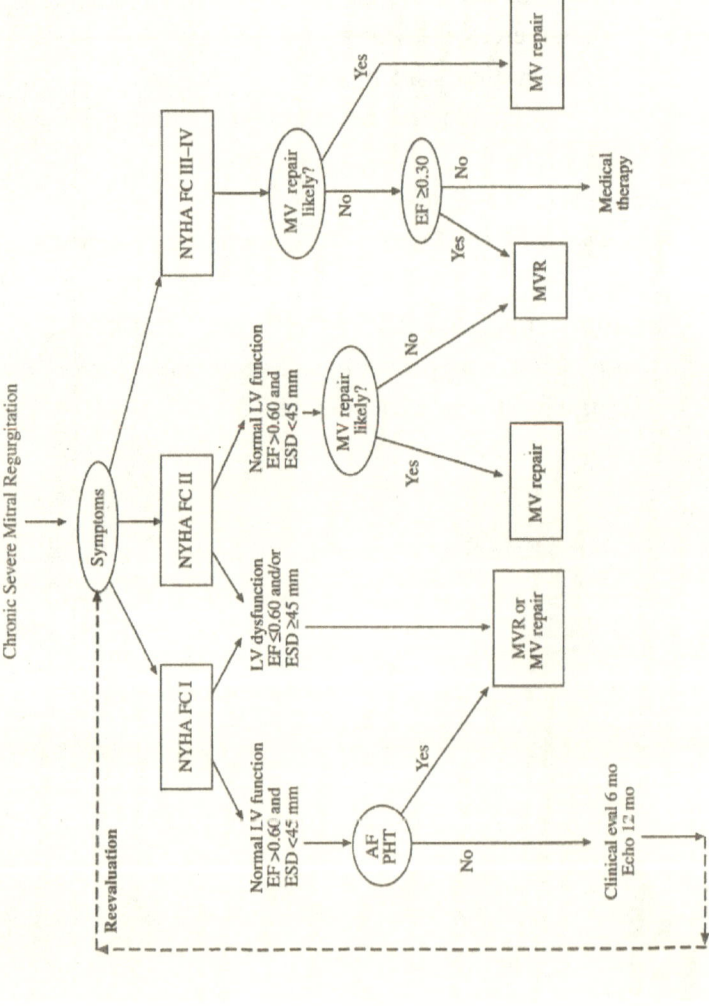

Chronic Severe Mitral Regurgitation

JACC 1998; Vol 32, No 5:1486-588

# Suggested Reading

1. Chapter 66: Valvular Heart Disease. Braunwald's Heart Disease(Elsevier), 9th ed., 1468-1539.

2. Chapter 2: Mitral Stenosis. Valvular Heart Disease. Edited by Dalen and Alpert (Little, brown and company). 2nd ed., 49-110

3. Chapter 3: Chronic Mitral Regurgitation. Valvular Heart Disease. Edited by Dalen and Alpert (Little, brown and company). 2nd ed., 111-150

4. Rapaport E: Calculation of valve areas. Eur Heart J 1985; 6 (suppl C): 21.

5. Clawson BJ. Rheumatic heart disease. An analysis of 796 cases. Am Heart J 1940;20:454–74

6. Kouchoukas NT, Blackstone EH, Doty DB *et al. Kirklin/Barratt-Boyes Cardiac Surgery. Morphology, diagnostic criteria, natural history, techniques, results and indications.* Churchill Livingstone, 3rd Edition, 2003

7. Rittoo D. Mitral Balloon Valvotomy. *B J Hosp Med* 1995;53:215-19

8. Inoue K, Owaki T, Nakamura T *et al.* Clinical application of transvenous mitral commissurotomy by a new balloon catheter. *J Thorac Cardiovasc Surg* 1984;87:394-402

9. Wilkins GT, Weymen AE, Abascal VM, Block PC, Palacios IF. Percutaneous balloon dilation of the mitral valve: an analysis of echocardiographic variables related to outcome and the mechanism of dilatation. Br Heart J. 1988;60:299-308.

10. Rapaport E. Natural history of aortic and mitral valve disease Am J Cardiol 1975;35:221-227

11. Fann JI, Ingels NB, Miller DC. Pathophysiology of Mitral Valve Disease. In: *Cardiac Surgery in the Adult.* 3rd ed. New York, NY: McGraw-Hill; 2008:chap 41.

12. Vahanian A, Alfieri O, Andreotti F, Antunes MJ, Barón-Esquivias G, Baumgartner H, et al. Guidelines on the management of valvular heart disease (version 2012): The Joint Task Force on the Management of Valvular Heart Disease of the European Society of Cardiology (ESC) and the European Association for Cardio-Thoracic Surgery (EACTS). *Eur Heart J.* Oct 2012;33(19):2451-96

13. Zoghbi WA, Enriquez-Sarano M, Foster E, et al: Recommendations

for evaluation of the severity of native valvular regurgitation with two-dimensional and Doppler echocardiography. J Am Soc Echocardiogr. 2003, 16: 777-802.

14. American College of Cardiology; American Heart Association Task Force on Practice Guidelines (Writing Committee to revise the 1998 guidelines for the management of patients with valvular heart disease); Society of Cardiovascular Anesthesiologists; Bonow RO, Carabello BA, Chatterjee K, et al: ACC/AHA 2006 guidelines for the management of patients with valvular heart disease. J Am Coll Cardiol. 2006, 48: e1-e148.

15. Bonow RO, Carabello BA, Chatterjee K, et al: 2006 Writing Committee Members; American College of Cardiology/American Heart Association Task Force. 2008 Focused update incorporated into the ACC/AHA 2006 guidelines for the management of patients with valvular heart disease: a report of the American College of Cardiology/American Heart Association Task Force on Practice Guidelines (Writing Committee to Revise the 1998 Guidelines for the Management of Patients With Valvular Heart Disease). Circulation. 2008, 118: e523-e661

# Abbreviations

| ACE: | Angiotensin converting enzyme |
| A2: | Aortic component of second heart sound |
| A2C: | Apical two chamber |
| A4C: | Apical four chamber |
| A5C: | Apical five chamber |
| AF: | Atrial fibrillation |
| AI: | Aortic insufficiency / Aortic incompetence |
| AO: | Aorta |
| AML: | Anterior mitral leaflet |
| AR: | Aortic regurgitation |
| ARF: | Acute rheumatic fever |
| AS: | Aortic stenosis |
| ASD: | Atrial septal defect |
| AV: | Aortic valve |
| AVG: | Aortic valve gradient |
| AVA: | Aortic valve area |
| AVR: | Aortic valve replacement |
| | |
| BB: | Beta blockers |
| BMV: | Balloon mitral valvotomy |
| BP: | Blood pressure |
| | |
| CABG: | Coronary artery bypass graft surgery |
| CAD: | Coronary artery disease |
| CCB: | Calcium channel blockers |
| CCF: | Congestive cardiac failure |
| CE: | Cardiac enlargement |
| CHB: | Complete heart block |
| CHF: | Congestive heart failure |
| CMC: | **Closed mitral commissurotomy** |
| CMV: | **Closed mitral valvotomy** |
| COPD: | Chronic obstructive pulmonary disease |
| CT: | Computed tomography |
| CTR: | Cardio thoracic ratio |
| CW: | Continuous wave |

| | |
|---|---|
| CXR: | Chest X-ray |
| | |
| DBP: | Diastolic blood pressure |
| D/D: | Differential diagnosis |
| DOE: | Dyspnea on exertion |
| | |
| EC: | Ejection click |
| ECG: | Electrocardiogram |
| EDM: | Early diastolic murmur |
| EF: | Ejection fraction |
| EI: | Eccentricity index |
| E/O: | Evidence of |
| ERO: | Effective regurgitant orifice |
| ESD: | End systolic diameter |
| ESM: | Ejection systolic murmur |
| ESS: | End systolic stress |
| ESV: | End systolic volume |
| ESVI: | End systolic volume index |
| | |
| F/U: | Follow up |
| Fr: | French |
| FS: | Fractional shortening |
| | |
| GI: | Gastrointestinal |
| | |
| HCM: | Hypertrophic cardiomyopathy |
| HOCM: | Hypertrophic obstructive cardiomyopathy |
| HT: | Hypertension |
| | |
| IAS: | Inter atrial septum |
| ICS: | Intercostal space |
| IE: | Infective endocarditis |
| IHJ: | Indian Heart Journal |
| IRBBB: | Incomplete right bundle branch block |
| IV: | Intra-venous |

| | |
|---|---|
| IVS: | Inter ventricular septum |
| JVP: | Jugular venous pulse |
| | |
| L → R: | Left to right |
| LA: | Left atrium |
| LAA: | Left atrial appendage |
| LAE: | Left atrial enlargement |
| LAP: | Left atrial pressure |
| LBBB: | Left bundle branch block |
| LICS: | Left intercostal space |
| LPA: | Left pulmonary artery |
| LSB: | Left sternal border |
| LV: | Left ventricle |
| LVEF: | Left ventricular ejection fraction |
| LVEDP: | Left ventricular end diastolic pressure |
| LVEDV: | Left ventricular end diastolic volume |
| LVEDVI: | Left ventricular end diastolic volume index |
| LVESV: | Left ventricular end systolic volume |
| LVESD: | Left ventricular end systolic diameter |
| LVESVI: | Left ventricular end systolic volume index |
| LVF: | Left ventricular failure |
| LVH: | Left ventricular hypertrophy |
| LVID: | LV internal diameter |
| LVIDS: | LV internal diameter in systole |
| LVIDD: | LV internal diameter in diastole |
| LVS3: | Left ventricular third heart sound |
| LVSP: | Left ventricular systolic pressure |
| LVOT: | Left ventricle outflow tract |
| LVOTO: | Left ventricle outflow tract obstruction |
| LVVO: | Left ventricular volume overload |
| | |
| MDM: | Mid diastolic murmur |
| MPA: | Main pulmonary artery |
| MR: | Mitral regurgitation |
| MS: | Mitral stenosis |

| | |
|---|---|
| MV: | Mitral valve |
| MVA: | Mitral valve area |
| MVD: | Mitral Valve disease |
| MVP: | Mitral valve prolapse |
| MVR: | Mitral valve replacement |
| | |
| NSR: | Normal sinus rhythm |
| NYHA: | New York Heart Association |
| | |
| O2: | Oxygen |
| **OMC:** | **Open mitral commissurotomy** |
| **OMV:** | **Open mitral valvotomy** |
| OS: | Opening snap |
| | |
| P2: | Pulmonary component of second heart sound |
| PA: | Pulmonary artery |
| PAP: | Pulmonary artery pressure |
| PAH: | Pulmonary arterial hypertension |
| PASP: | Pulmonary artery systolic pressure |
| *PAWP:* | *Pulmonary artery wedge pressure* |
| *PDA:* | *Patent ductus arteriosus* |
| PH: | Pulmonary hypertension |
| PHT: | Pressure half time |
| PISA: | Proximal Isovelocity Surface Area |
| *PLAX:* | *Parasternal long axis* |
| *PMD:* | Papillary muscle dysfunction |
| PML: | Posterior mitral leaflet |
| PND: | Paroxysmal nocturnal dyspnea |
| PR: | Pulmonary regurgitation |
| PSA: | Presystolic accentuation |
| *PSAX:* | *Parasternal short axis* |
| *PSM:* | *Pansystolic murmur* |
| PTMC: | Percutaneous transvenous mitral commissurotomy |
| PTMV: | Percutaneous mitral balloon valvotomy |
| *PV:* | *Pulmonary valve* |

| | |
|---|---|
| *PVOD:* | *Pulmonary vascular obstructive disease* |
| PW: | Pulse wave |
| | |
| RA: | Right atrium |
| RAE: | Right atrial enlargement |
| RAP: | Right atrial pressure |
| RF: | Regurgitant fraction |
| RF: | Rheumatic fever |
| RHD: | Rheumatic heart disease |
| RHF: | Right heart failure |
| RICS: | Right intercostal space |
| RPA: | Right pulmonary artery |
| RV: | Right ventricle |
| RV: | Regurgitant volume |
| RVE: | Right ventricular enlargement |
| RVEDP: | Right ventricular end diastolic pressure |
| RVF: | Right ventricular failure |
| RVH: | Right ventricular hypertrophy |
| RVOT: | Right ventricle outflow tract |
| RVSP: | Right ventricular systolic pressure |
| RVS3: | Right ventricular third heart sound |
| RVS4: | Right ventricular fourth heart sound |
| Rx: | Treatment |
| | |
| S1: | First heart sound |
| S2: | Second heart sound |
| S3: | Third heart sound |
| S4: | Fourth heart sound |
| *SAM:* | *Systolic anterior motion* |
| SBP: | Systolic blood pressure |
| *SCD:* | Sudden cardiac death |
| SLE: | Systemic lupus erythematosus |
| *SM:* | *Systolic murmur* |
| STS: | Society of Thoracic Surgeons |
| SV: | Stroke volume |

| | |
|---|---|
| TEE: | Trans esophageal echocardiography |
| TIA: | Transient ischemic attack |
| TGA: | Transposition of great arteries |
| TMG: | Transmitral gradient |
| TMT: | Treadmill test |
| TOF: | Tetralogy Of Fallot |
| TTE: | Trans thoracic echocardiography |
| TR: | Tricuspid regurgitation |
| TS: | Tricuspid stenosis |
| TV: | Tricuspid valve |
| | |
| Va: | Aliasing velocity |
| VCW: | Vena contracta width |
| VACA: | Valvuloplasty and Angioplasty in Congenital Anomalies |
| VSD: | Ventricular septal defect |
| VTI: | Velocity time integral |